Say Stop to A[illegible] and Depression

Yes….now you can….Recover and Regain Control of your Life – Rewire your Mind and Start Living – Overcome Panic and Anger. A Self Help Guide……

Jonathan Douglas

rendering of legal, financial, medical or professional advice. The content within this book has been derived from various sources. Please consult a licensed professional before attempting any techniques outlined in this book.

By reading this document, the reader agrees that under no circumstances is the author responsible for any losses, direct or indirect, that are incurred as a result of the use of information contained within this document, including, but not limited to, errors, omissions, or inaccuracies.

Table of Contents

Table of Contents

Introduction...*8*

Chapter 1: Understanding Anxiety............................*11*

What is Anxiety?..**12**

Worry vs. Anxiety..13

Determining Your Anxiety Level.....................................15

Signs and Symptoms of Anxiety......................................17

Causes of Anxiety..**21**

Types of Anxiety Disorders.....................................**23**

Generalized Anxiety Disorder...23

Panic Disorder...25

Phobias..26

Selective Mutism..30

Obsessive-Compulsive Disorder.....................................33

Separation Anxiety Disorder..35

Post-Traumatic Stress Disorder......................................37

Chapter 2: Your Thoughts and Your State of Being.40

Manage Your Anxiety by Managing Your Thoughts42

Understanding Your Emotions and Feelings...................42

How to Avoid Anxious Thoughts....................................45

Face the Thought...46

Create or Choose a Different Thought...........................53

Write Out the Thought and Worry About It Later............56

Solvable and Unsolvable Worries..........................59

Negative Self-Talk = Self Destruction......................61

Stop Letting Your Past Define You..................................62

Halting Negative Self-Talk..63

Chapter 3: Exercises for Managing Anxiety............69

Sympathetic Nervous System vs. Parasympathetic Nervous System...69

Mindfulness Exercises..74

Benefits of Mindfulness..75

Suggested Mindfulness Exercises....................................76

Meditation Exercises..80

Suggested Meditation Practice to Decrease Anxiety.........81

What If You Just Can't Practice Meditation?...................83

Breathing Exercises...84

Suggested Breathing Exercise for Relaxation..................86

Exercise Therapy...90

Yoga...91

Ways to Find Instant Calm......................................94

Positive Self-Talk...95

Guided Imagery...97

Tips...100

Practice Gratitude...100

Touching Your Lips...105

Creativity and Hobbies..107

Chapter 4: Managing Your Time, Energy, and Activities...109

Fretting About Time Management vs. Designing Your Day......109

Prune Your Daily To-Do List......110

Create Three Lists......112

Group Your Daily Tasks into Batches of Similar Tasks...112

Recognize the Difference between Important and Urgent Tasks......113

Focus on Your Plans, Not Other's......114

Create Time for Focused Work......115

Learn to Keep a Schedule......116

Stay Calm If Things Pop Up......117

Find Out Where You Are Spending Your Time......118

Make Time for Yourself......119

Chapter 5: Therapeutic and Clinical Treatment......121

Therapy......121

The Self-Option CBT Guidelines......123

Changing Your Lifestyle to Regain Control of Your Life......124

Cognitive Techniques......124

Behavioral Techniques......125

Quality Sleep Decreases Worry and Anxiety......126

Medication for Anxiety and Panic Attacks......129

Questions to Ask Yourself......134

Questions to Ask Your Doctor......135

Herbal Supplements for Treating Anxiety......135

Conclusion......138

References...141

Introduction

Modernization makes us believe that we live in a world where everything has to be fast-paced. When things don't happen as fast as we think they should, we start to worry. We worry that money isn't coming in as expected and that the bills are piling up! We are anxious that the kids aren't behaving well, and they'll soon grow into young adults where it'll be difficult to mold them. We are afraid for our health and fitness because the results of the diets and workouts aren't showing quick enough. We are not sure if our spouses will stick with us for the long haul, so we fret about the unknown future. The list seems to be endless.

Many people almost fall asleep ruminating on all the many things bothering them. This puts their mind and body in a continuous tensed state waiting for the proverbial last straw that would break the camel's back. Little wonder a lot of people suffer from one or more forms of anxiety disorder. When our minds and bodies are constantly preparing for threats to our survival (and in many cases, these threats are not real but merely perceived ones), our body's defense system weakens over time, making us susceptible to mental health disorders.

Worrisome thoughts may feel like the only place where we can turn to and find solace, but the fact is, they don't make our situations any better. If anything, they cause us more psychological and physiological problems. But it isn't that most of us don't know the negative impacts of worry on our mental and physical health; it's just that a lot of us don't know how to manage, reduce, or even avoid these anxious thoughts altogether.

To keep worrisome thoughts at bay with its associated unpleasant physical symptoms, I have outlined several simple but effective techniques that you can begin to implement right away. Some of these techniques can be used anywhere and they don't take much of your time. The techniques work; however, they do not eliminate your anxiety overnight. As much as I would like to show you a trick that you can wave like a magic wand to make all your worries go away at once, the fact remains that no such scientifically proven tips, tricks, techniques or magic exist – at least, for now. Your worries and anxieties will lose their grip on you if you consistently practice the techniques described in this book. You will need to give the methods as well as yourself time and learn to be patient with yourself.

Of course, you have the option of getting clinical treatment for anxiety disorders – and I strongly recommend that you pursue that option if your anxiety has become a mental health disorder. You will also find a short guide on the type of therapy to use, should you opt for that.

If anxiety has taken its toll on your physical and mental health, you will find in the pages of this book, some of the quickest routes to your recovery! I strongly urge you to put into practice what you are about to learn.

Here is to your success and quick recovery.

Jonathan Douglas

Chapter 1: Understanding Anxiety

We all have some level of worry and anxiety; that is a given. Anxiety is our body's natural way of reacting to stress – telling us that something is out of place or something may go wrong so that we can focus our energies on dealing with the source of the stress. Under normal circumstances, anxiety is a healthy emotion. A little bit of worry from time to time can be advantageous. For example, when meeting your would-be in-laws for the first time, when you have an upcoming job interview, test, or exam, and when you have to make a business presentation to the board of directors in your organization. It is natural for you to become anxious and even worry a bit about these situations. But the result of this worry can be positive because it can push you to prepare yourself well ahead of time to give a good first impression to your future in-laws, prepare well for the interview, test, or exam, or get your act together to deliver an impressive business presentation. In other words, the fear of embarrassing yourself in a stressful situation has pushed you to take action to better handle the situation and properly deal with the source of anxiety. In this regard, worry and anxiety serve a positive purpose.

Nevertheless, anxiety becomes a problem if it is a constant fixture in our lives. If worrying becomes a habit, it can lead to serious damages and could indicate an underlying disorder problem such as social anxiety, panic disorder, or generalized anxiety disorder. To understand the type of anxiety this book deals with and to know when you are stepping beyond the normal levels of anxiety, let us briefly take a look at some key definitions.

What is Anxiety?

According to the American Psychological Association (APA), "Anxiety is an emotion characterized by feelings of tension, worried thoughts and physical changes like increased blood pressure" (American Psychological Association, 2019).

When thoughts of fear and worry begin to negatively affect your daily activities, your anxiety level is gradually tilting towards a mental health disorder. As earlier mentioned, anxiety is a natural reaction to stressful situations; it is how our body is designed to respond to threats whether they are real or perceived. Our bodies receive a series of signals from our brains when we perceived any threat to fight (defend ourselves) or take flight (protect ourselves). This natural threat-response system causes us to experience anxiety. Some of the symptoms of anxiety include fast heart rate, shortness of breath or rapid breathing, and excessive worry.

Worry vs. Anxiety

But is anxiety the same as worry? How do you know if what you have is anxiety or worry? And how do you know if your anxiety level is okay or you are beginning to tilt towards a problematic level of anxiety?

Even though worry and anxiety are used interchangeably, worry is just one out of the three major constituents of anxiety. The three major constituents of anxiety are cognitive, physiological, and emotional problems. Let us assume that you are expected to give a speech at one of your company's event. On hearing that, your thoughts immediately bring up all the eyes that will be on you as you stand on the podium and you start to think of how you are such a bad speaker and how everyone will see your flaws. This unwanted thought causes you to think you can't handle the task of public speaking. This unwanted or negative thought is what worry is, and it is the cognitive component of anxiety. As a result of worrying, you may begin to feel dreadful and fearful about the event. This is the emotional component of anxiety playing out. The physiological components are represented by bodily sensations, like sweating, rapid heart rate, and a sudden tightness in your stomach.

One of the clearest indications that your anxiety level is getting out of hand is an increase in difficulty in doing things that you once found relatively easy. This could be having an intense fear of public speaking, being unable to ride in an elevator, doing everything possible to avoid meeting new people, and so on. Once you notice that your anxious feelings are beginning to get in the way of your daily living (taking the stairs in a 10-story building instead of taking an elevator!) you need to take immediate steps to get your life back.

Other ways to know that your anxiety level is becoming problematic include:

- Worry tends to be associated with known facts, which makes it a lot easier to look for practical solutions towards handling the worry. Anxiety tends to be based on beliefs and can sometimes be vague. It is difficult to find a solution to something you can't put a finger on, which is why anxiety is a prolonged form of unchecked worry.

- Intense anxiety shows up in a consistent feeling of fear, sadness, or guilt, as opposed to temporal worry that is related to a specific situation. With everyday worry, you can take action to resolve the specific situation that is causing the worry, but with problematic anxiety, the feeling is persistent, and there seems to be no definite action that can immediately resolve it.

- Safe levels of worry usually end up only in your head as unwanted thoughts. For example, "I can't pass the test," "I'll probably make a fool of myself in front of all those people." These thoughts can be replaced by something more helpful. Anxiety disorder, on the other hand, is accompanied by intense emotional and physiological responses in addition to persistent worry.

- You can perform optimally even when you have regular worries; it does not interfere with your everyday functions. Anxiety is intense and is capable of disrupting your sleep, social life, work, relationships, and even your appetite.

The above distinction notwithstanding, I shall use the terms "worry" and "anxiety" interchangeably in some parts of this book. The distinction was to provide clarity and to help you know when to seek help.

Determining Your Anxiety Level

Generally, when a stressful situation is encountered, anxiety is experienced. But when the anxious feeling gets out of proportion to the stressful situation or the trigger, it shows that the individual has gone beyond normal anxiety levels and is showing signs of anxiety disorder – a situation where concerns and intrusive thoughts are a recurring and dominant theme in the individual's life.

So, on one end of the anxiety spectrum, there is the everyday mild anxiety and worry, which can be referred to as the helpful side of anxiety and worry. On the other end of the spectrum, there is the problematic or clinical anxiety disorder, which is unhelpful because it can cause impairment to normal functions.

But there is also a midpoint where an individual is not experiencing a full-blown anxiety disorder even though they have gone beyond the normal feeling of temporal anxiety. According to Luana Marques, Ph.D., writing for Harvard Medical School, states that, "When the level of anxiety you experience is no longer adaptive or helpful to your performance and becomes a barrier to your enjoyment of life, but does not yet meet the diagnostic threshold for an anxiety disorder, you are 'almost anxious'" (Marques, 2018).

This means that there three levels in which you can experience anxiety: the normal mild anxiety level, the midpoint or "almost anxious" level, and the clinical anxiety level, which is known as an anxiety disorder.

To illustrate the different levels of anxiety, imagine that Howard, a midlevel manager, is experiencing the first (normal) anxiety level. He goes to work, worries about things, fears some tasks, but still performs his normal functions. If Howard experiences the second (almost anxious) level, he can still get to work but will spend a large chunk of his working hours staring into space and getting just a few tasks done. He can still perform some tasks but is mostly distracted by debilitating thoughts and feels unpleasant sensations like a tight chest, upset stomach, and racing heart. Although Howard was not held back at home by anxiety, he still can't function optimally at work because of the level of anxiety he is experiencing. If Howard is attuned to himself, he would begin seeking help at this point before he slips into the third level. On the third level, Howard may likely avoid work for several days in a row because he is having a panic attack. This is a full-blown anxiety disorder.

Signs and Symptoms of Anxiety

Apart from cowering in his room for several days in a row because of a panic attack, here some signs and symptoms for Howard (and those like him) to know if he is having some form of anxiety disorder. Note that there are several diagnoses for anxiety disorders and each type has its specific symptoms; however, the common symptoms are given below.

1. **Too much worrying**: Excessive worrying is one of the topmost symptoms of an anxiety disorder. When you worry too much, usually in disproportionate amounts to

any given situation and for a considerable period, it could mean you are having an anxiety disorder. When worrisome thoughts make it very difficult for you to concentrate and stop you from getting things done, you are showing signs that your worries are difficult to control – a clear sign of anxiety disorder.

2. **Having a strong need to avoid social situations**: One form of anxiety disorder is known as a social anxiety disorder. It can show up as:

    - A fear of being judged and humiliated or looked down by others.
    - Feeling dreadful about an upcoming social situation.
    - Worrying about embarrassing yourself in front of others.
    - Shunning social situations and events to stay protected from public glare.

    This can make the individual appear very quiet and shy when meeting new people or when in a group. A person with a social anxiety disorder may appear calm on the outside but experience uncomfortable turbulence inwardly. Social anxiety disorder could be the result of low self-esteem, depression, or even harsh self-criticism and can make the individual appear snobbish.

3. **Feeling restless or being on-edge**: Feeling jumpy, uneasy, and nervous most of the time is a sign of anxiety disorder. This happens because your brain thinks that you are in some sort of danger, and it is preparing your body to respond to the threat. In other words, your sympathetic nervous system has shifted its gears into overdrive in readiness for a fight-or-flight response. When this occurs, you may experience dry mouth, sweaty palms, shaky hands, and a racy pulse. This is all good if there is an actual danger. But if the fear is all in your head, it could be a debilitating experience. Blood moves from your digestive system to your muscles preparing you for defense or protection, your senses are heightened to make you more aware of your environment. But the fight-or-flight never really happens – your body simply continues in a state of readiness for a physical activity that doesn't happen (Hoehn-Saric and McLeod, 2000).

4. **Sleep disturbances**: When you have trouble falling asleep or staying asleep, it could be a sign of an anxiety disorder. Insomnia and anxiety disorder are closely linked, even though it is not clear which leads to the other or if both contribute to each other (National Institute of Health, 2008). However, when an anxiety disorder is treated, it usually improves sleep quality.

5. **Extreme irrational fears**: Irrational fears can be a sign of an anxiety disorder. When you have extreme fears about certain situations or objects such as heights, open spaces, enclosed spaces, or animals, and the fear of these things interferes with your ability to function normally, it could be a sign of an anxiety disorder.

6. **Intense physiological responses**: Recurring intense physiological responses such as shortness of breath, nausea, sweating, and the fear of losing control or dying could be an indication of anxiety disorder, especially when they are accompanied by an intense feeling of fear.

7. **Tense muscles**: As with the case of insomnia, tense muscles are associated with anxiety disorders especially when they are experienced for a prolonged period. Treating tense muscles can greatly improve symptoms of anxiety disorder.

8. **Excessive touchiness**: People with a generalized anxiety disorder are known to be very touchy, especially during the peak of their anxiety disorder, according to a study that included over 6,000 adult participants (National Institute of Health, 2017). Excessive touchiness should be expected given that the anxiety disorder is associated with excessive worrisome thoughts. In a mental state of worry, it is easy to become highly irritable.

9. **Frequent fatigue**: Anxiety is usually associated with arousal and hyperactivity, so it may come as a surprise to see frequent fatigue as one of the symptoms of anxiety disorders. Fatigue alone is not a clear indicator of an anxiety disorder as fatigue can also be linked to depression or other medical conditions. However, it is important to note that a chronic feeling of fatigue especially after an anxiety attack can be a pointer to anxiety disorders. Fatigue can also be a result of hormonal effects due to persistent anxiety, muscle tension, or insomnia.

Causes of Anxiety

So, what exactly causes us to be so anxious to the point that it becomes a disorder? Well, it may be difficult to point out just one cause of anxiety disorders because causes can be multifaceted a lot of the time. Let us consider a few of these factors.

1. Medical factors – The side effect of medications can cause anxiety just like an underlying disease would. People who have heart conditions, asthma attacks, or anemia, among other conditions, can experience symptoms of anxiety

disorders. Prescription medication for asthma, thyroid, and over-the-counter decongestants can also add to anxiety.

2. Heredity – It is possible for people whose family members suffer from anxiety disorders to experience such disorders themselves.

3. Stress – This is one of the major causes of anxiety disorders especially in a modern world full of stress-inducing activities. Stress could be in the form of financial pressures, academics, relationships and family drama, and work-related.

4. Brain chemistry – Traumatic experiences such as head trauma or brain tumor can greatly affect brain structure and function.

5. Use of substances or withdrawal from substances – When combined with the stress of daily living, illicit substances can contribute to anxiety disorders. Also, an attempt to withdraw from their use can equally contribute to increasing the level of the individual's anxiety. People who are already experiencing some form of anxiety disorder may also find that consuming caffeine increases nervousness and makes them jittery. Caffeine is a stimulant that affects your fight-or-flight response

system. Consuming caffeine is likely to keep someone with an anxiety disorder up for most of the night.

6. Environment – Certain environments can trigger anxiety. For example, symptoms of anxiety can be experienced in high-altitude areas where there is a low oxygen level.

Any of the above factors or a combination of two or more factors can result in anxiety disorder. For example, taking illicit substances to temporary douse the tension of an abusive relationship, a traumatic experience like the loss of a loved one, or to lessen the burden of work-related pressure can increase anxiety levels and may likely lead to more complications.

Types of Anxiety Disorders

When anxiety becomes a recurring feeling and coupled with intrusive concerns or thoughts, it is a disorder. Although anxiety disorders have some common signs and symptoms, their diagnosis and impacts on the individual's health and daily functions differ as shown in this section.

Generalized Anxiety Disorder

Do you feel as if something is off but you just can't put a finger on it even though you can't seem to shake that feeling? You're not alone. Generalized anxiety disorder (GAD) is one of the most common types of anxiety disorder suffered by a lot of people. For many people, it is a bit tricky to identify the source or cause of their anxiety – they simply "know" that something is not as it should be, which keeps them in a continuous state of worry. GAD can interfere with a person's normal sleep time and can also cause them to lose appetite. Worrisome thoughts associated with GAD can lead to a loss of concentration and a depletion of energy.

Symptoms of GAD are:

- An unrealistic and often illogical perspective on problems.
- Difficulty in falling or staying asleep.
- Easily startled.
- Finding it difficult to concentrate.
- Having a frequent need to go to the bathroom.
- Headaches.

- Muscle tension.
- Nausea.
- Restlessness.
- Sweating.
- Touchiness.
- Trembling.
- Unnecessary, ongoing worry.

Panic Disorder

A person who suffers brief moments of intense terror and apprehension is showing signs of a panic disorder. These panic attacks often lead to nausea, dizziness, shortness of breath or difficulty in breathing, palpitations, shaking, and confusion. If not treated, panic attacks can escalate very quickly. Usually, those who suffer this type of anxiety disorder have been exposed to prolonged stress or have had some very frightening experience. Nevertheless, a panic attack can also occur without an obvious trigger. Sometimes, a person who experiences a panic attack may feel disconnected from reality – a condition known as derealization. His or her mind may go completely blank as if they are detached from themselves and are merely experiencing themselves from a place outside of themselves. People who suffer panic disorder may withdraw from family and friends due to the fear of a recurrence. If left untreated, it is capable of severely disrupting a person's quality of life.

Since other medical conditions such as an overactive thyroid, heart abnormalities, and even caffeine consumption can have the same symptoms as a panic disorder, a single episode of a panic attack may not qualify as an anxiety disorder. The individual with the condition would have experienced these attacks repeatedly for it to qualify as a panic disorder.

Phobias

A phobia is an extreme and usually illogical aversion to something or a fear of a situation, place, object, or a living creature. People who have phobias will go to great lengths in shaping their lives to avoid their phobias. How they picture the threat is a lot greater than the actual threat posed by what they fear. A person with a phobia can experience panic attacks due to the intense nature of the distress they feel when faced with their fears. Phobias are categorized into three main types. They are:

1. **Social anxiety or social phobia**: This is having a heightened sense of fear about being negatively judged by others in a social situation. It is also the fear of public

embarrassment. Of course, no one wants to experience public embarrassment or enjoys being judged negatively by others, but a person who suffers from social anxiety disorder will make his decisions based on the possibility of these negative responses. In other words, if the person perceives that a situation can potentially put him or her in a position that they will be criticized or embarrassed, they will do all they can to avoid such a situation. A person who doesn't have this disorder would prepare better for the situation or take it in their strides. People who have this type of anxiety disorder may also experience a range of feelings such as fear of being rejected, stage fright, and intense doubts about intimacy. Social anxiety disorder can deprive the sufferer of enjoying human contact and the benefits of actively participating in groups.

2. **Agoraphobia**: This is an anxiety disorder that shows up as extreme fear of situations, events, and places where help might not be readily available or where escape would be difficult in the event of a mishap. Many people who develop agoraphobia have experienced panic attacks one or more times. To avoid further panic attacks, they would do all they can to avoid places, situations, and events that trigger such attacks. The triggers could be crowds, elevators, public transport, air travel, open spaces, and

remote areas. A person with agoraphobia may require the help of a companion to cope in these situations and places. Sometimes, people with agoraphobia may find it difficult to leave home for fear of a panic attack. Agoraphobia can greatly impair the wellbeing of an individual because it is a complex phobia. A person who has the disorder usually experiences other types of phobias. For example, a person who has a fear of being left alone (monophobia) is likely to also have a fear of being trapped in closed spaces (claustrophobia).

3. **Specific phobia**: This is extreme fear and avoidance of a specific trigger. The trigger could be an animal (such as snakes and spiders), a place (such as being on an airplane, on a tall building, on a bridge, or in a tunnel), or a situation (such as in a crowd). Specific phobias usually develop early in an individual's life. In some cases, a traumatic experience during the formative ages will lead to such fears over the years. In some other cases, a child that witnesses his or her parent or a family member experience intense fear for a specific object, situation, or place may also develop such fears over time. Specific phobias are not complex; they can be traced to a specific cause and have a less negative impact on the overall wellbeing of the individual because the trigger may not be a common occurrence in everyday life. For example, a

person with the fear of snakes may not see snakes every day, therefore, he or she can function normally unless on the rare occasion where snakes are encountered.

People with phobias may acknowledge that their fear is very irrational, but because it is a disorder, they feel very helpless to control their extreme feeling of fear when they are exposed to their triggers. Phobias can be very illogical to a person who doesn't have them, but to the sufferer, it can evoke such intense feeling as to disrupt normal function. Some common phobias include:

- Fear of heights (acrophobia)
- Fear of flying (aerophobia)
- Fear of water (aquaphobia)
- Fear of spiders (arachnophobia)
- Fear of confined spaces (claustrophobia)
- Fear of vomiting (emetophobia)
- Fear of blushing (erythrophobia)
- Fear of escalators (escalaphobia)
- Fear of becoming ill (hypochondria)

- Fear of tunnels (tunnel phobia)
- Fear of animals (zoophobia)

The list of phobias continues to grow as society changes because people can develop a phobia of just about anything. For example, recently a paper describes nomophobia as "the pathologic fear of remaining out of touch with technology" (King et al., 2010). People now have a fear of being without their computers and cell phones! We never can tell what phobia will crop up next.

Selective Mutism

Selective mutism is an anxiety disorder that starts during childhood. If a child has excellent verbal communication when he or she is with family, friends, and familiar people but tends to go mute in certain settings, such as in school and other public places, the child likely has selective mutism. This type of disorder may be an extreme form of social anxiety. It is an intense feeling of panic that comes along with a freeze response when in certain situations that the child is expected to speak. If left untreated, selective mutism can persist into adulthood (NHS, 2019).

It is important to note the following about selective mutism:

- The child or person with selective mutism does not deliberately refuse to speak in certain settings or situations. They are literally incapable of speaking (temporarily).

- Selective mutism is not the same as merely being shy. It is an anxiety disorder.

- The disturbance is not as a result of stuttering and other forms of speech or communication disorder.

- For the disturbance to qualify as selective mutism it must be shown to interfere with learning, social communication, or occupational achievement.

- Also, before a child can be said to have selective mutism, he or she would have to have experienced the disorder for at least a month. This period should not be limited to when the child is in a new environment, such as in their first month of school.

- When a child is unable to speak due to a language barrier or a lack of knowledge in what is being discussed, it doesn't count as selective mutism.

- A person who is unable to speak due to some psychotic or developmental disorder cannot be said to have selective mutism.

How can you tell if your child has selective mutism and is not just being shy? Selective mutism starts to manifest early in childhood, usually between the ages of 2 and 4. It can be observed when the child starts to be exposed to other people outside their family such as classmates, teachers, unfamiliar relatives, and other adults.

Here are the common signs to know if your child has selective mutism:

- They have a sudden frozen facial expression and stillness about them when they are expected to speak in certain settings or to certain people.

- They avoid eye contact and appear very uneasy, nervous, and behave awkwardly in social settings.

- The child becomes extremely shy and withdrawn in situations where he or she is expected to fully participate.

- They become unnecessarily clingy, sulky, disinterested, and rude.

- When prompted to speak, they become poorly coordinated, tense, and stiff.

Children with selective mutism who are a bit confident may respond to communication with gestures. For example, a child can nod or shake their head for "yes" and "no," respectively.

Some children may simply respond with an altered voice such as whispering or they may manage to utter few words. In other children with severe cases of selective mutism, communication in written, spoken, or gestured forms is completely avoided when they experience their trigger.

If a child begins to show any of these signs, it is advisable to take proper steps to get help to stop the disorder from persisting into adulthood. Don't assume that they will grow out of it or that they are just being shy. That could be a very costly assumption.

Obsessive-Compulsive Disorder

Do you know of someone who seems to be obsessed

about the way things are arranged or who seems to always double checks and even triple check things just to be sure? Such a person may be showing signs of Obsessive-Compulsive Disorder (OCD). OCD is a chronic disorder in which the individual continues to have recurring thoughts (obsession) and irresistible behaviors (compulsion) that tends to be repeated over and over. Performing rituals or double-checking things on their own may not point to OCD. In fact, they can make a person more focused and have a proper structure that makes their tasks a lot easier. However, a person with OCD experiences great distress if they do not follow their unwanted routines and behaviors.

A person with OCD:

- Is usually not able to control their thoughts and behaviors whether or not they acknowledge them to be excessive.
- Is exposed to problems in their daily activities as a direct result of their obsessive thoughts and compulsive behaviors.
- Spends an inordinate amount of time on these intrusive thoughts or behaviors.
- Only experiences a very brief relief from the anxiety that is caused by their intrusive thoughts but does not truly enjoy the obsessive thoughts or compulsive behavior.

A person with OCD may show signs and symptoms of obsession, compulsion, or both. These symptoms can get in the way of the individual's personal relationships, work, and school.

A person who has repeated intrusive thoughts or someone who experiences distressing mental images quite often may be suffering from obsession. The common symptoms of obsession include:

- Uncontrollable worry about contamination, harm, or germs.

- Unwanted thoughts involving religion and sex.
- A need to have things in symmetrical order or a need for exactness.
- Violent thoughts toward oneself or others.

Compulsion, on the other hand, is repetitive behavior in response to obsessive thoughts. The person with a compulsion feels a very strong urge to behave a certain way even when they know that the behavior is not necessary. The common symptoms of compulsion include:

- Compulsive counting of items.
- A strong need to avoid walking on cracks.
- Excessive need to clean or wash hands.
- Repeatedly checking things to make sure they are as should be. For example, checking to make sure that the oven is off or that the door is locked.
- Irresistible urge to have things arranged in a particular order.

Separation Anxiety Disorder

This is an anxiety disorder that is associated with children and young adolescents. When a child responds extremely terrified to separation or anticipated separation from his or her parent or caregiver, that child may be showing signs of separation anxiety disorder. The child may be separated from his or her attachment figure (primary caregiver) because they have to go to school or they have to go to bed at night. Under normal circumstances, symptoms of separation anxiety decline and resolve after a few weeks as the child gradually adjusts to the absence of his or her primary caregiver. But in some uncommon cases, the anxiety doesn't resolve; instead, it grows worse with time. So, instead of the child getting used to being without his or her primary caregiver, they grow clingier and experience greater distress when separated from their primary caregiver. Separation anxiety can negatively impact a child's academic performance. Also, children who are excessively terrified early in life have a greater likelihood of developing anxiety disorders that can lead to considerable impairment.

Here are some symptoms that indicate separation anxiety disorder:

- Reluctance to fall asleep in the absence of the primary caregiver.
- Nightmares (especially when they have separation-related themes).

- Homesickness.
- Irrational concerns for the safety of loved ones.
- Excessive tantrums in anticipation of separation from the primary caregiver.
- Psychosomatic symptoms such as dizziness, vomiting, headache, muscle aches, lightheadedness, cramps, stomach ache, nausea, and heart palpitations.

Post-Traumatic Stress Disorder

A person who witnessed or experienced a traumatic event, such as rape, violent death, a terrible accident, a natural disaster, or war, can develop Post-Traumatic Stress Disorder (PTSD). People who endure traumatic events may experience nightmares, flashbacks, severe anxiety, and intrusive thoughts about the event. But with adequate care and sufficient time, they can adjust, cope, and get better. However, if these symptoms persist over several months or years, and are a source of impairment to daily functioning, the individual may have PTSD.

A person with PTSD can exhibit any or all of the following four categories of PTSD symptoms in varying degrees:

1. **Intrusive memories**: This occurs in the form of

involuntary memories of the traumatic event. These memories can be so vivid that the person with PTSD will feel as if the event is happening all over again. This can bring back all the uncomfortable feelings associated with the traumatic event. A patient can also experience:

- Actual physical reactions and severe emotional distress in response to intrusive memories.
- Unwanted, uncontrollable, and recurrent memories of the traumatic event.
- Upsetting dreams related to the traumatic event.

2. **Avoidance**: This involves resisting thoughts of the traumatic event. A person with PTSD may try to live in denial of the traumatic event and try to suppress or not talk about how they feel about the event. They simply don't want to process the event for fear of reigniting the horrifying anxiety they experienced or witnessed during the event. This can make them:

   - Do everything possible to avoid talking or thinking about the traumatic event.
   - Deliberately avoid activities, places, people, situations, objects, and anything that can rekindle the memory of the traumatic event.

3. **Negative thinking and feelings**: This is an ongoing

negative and distorted belief about others and oneself. For example, "People cannot be trusted" or "I am not good enough." This can also affect how the individual views his or her future. Usually, PTSD can make one hopeless about the future. Other symptoms under this category include:

- Unable to let oneself experience positive emotions.
- Having a hard time maintaining close relationships.
- Feeling estranged from friends and family.
- Ongoing feeling of fear, guilt, horror, and being emotionally numb.
- Lacking interest in activities previously enjoyed.

4. **Changes in emotional and physical reactions (arousal symptoms)**: This is being easily aroused to physical and emotional reactions, such as angry outbursts and behaving in a self-destructive, aggressive, and reckless way. It can also include:

    - Always being on the lookout for threats.
    - Being easily frightened or startled.
    - Difficulty in concentrating.
    - Difficulty in sleeping.

Chapter 2: Your Thoughts and Your State of Being

Sometimes it can be annoying when you hear or read statements that seem to put the blame on you for how you feel. One such statement is, "All events are neutral; your interpretation of the event determines how you react or respond to it." Although it may not be a welcomed perspective (depending on your mood), it is still valid; your state of being, that is, how you feel, depends to a large extent on the types of thoughts you think about an event.

For example, two people (let's call them Adam and Joe) are in an elevator that suddenly stopped working. They realized that they are trapped and could be in the elevator for a while. Adam recalls several movie scenes where people got trapped in the elevator and something bad happened to them. He begins to think frantic thoughts and starts to panic. He kept pressing the buttons on the panel, banging the door, and screaming in the hope that someone would hear him. He was going hysterical and tiring himself in the process. Joe, on the other hand, was thinking of how great his business presentation went and didn't bother about the elevator. He didn't like being trapped in an elevator, but he knew that in all likelihood, someone was working on getting the elevator back to normal since Adam had pressed the call button. Joe tries to speak calmly to Adam, but Adam won't have any of that. After about 5 minutes, Joe pulls out his cell phone, calls his boss on one of the floors of the building, and informs him of the elevator problem. Only then did Adam realize he also had a cell phone on him. A couple of minutes later, they were both out of the elevator.

This may be a simple example, but it shows how two people can interpret and react differently to the same event because of the thoughts they choose to have about the event. Extreme feelings of anxiousness that can lead to irrational behaviors can be controlled if you can get a handle on your thinking process. Thinking negatively or in an unhelpful way will only increase worry and anxiety; shifting your thoughts to a more empowering one can significantly reduce anxiety.

However, you cannot possibly change a negative thought by merely changing "I am bad" into "I am good." If that were the case, nearly everyone could simply think their anxiety disorder out of existence! Trying to force yourself into thinking positive thoughts is not an authentic way to live and certainly not very helpful, especially if you suffer any mental health condition or live with any anxiety disorder. When practiced consistently, healthy thinking can improve anxiety and get rid of excessive worrying. But that may not be the case for everyone. The tips and techniques recommended in this book are not meant to dissuade you from getting professional help. If you find yourself stuck in a pattern of negative thoughts that won't go away, seek the help of a mental health professional as quickly as possible.

Manage Your Anxiety by Managing Your Thoughts

The feeling of anxiety is tied to your thoughts. If you can successfully manage your thought patterns, you can keep anxiety to a healthy level. It takes time and dedicated effort to achieve this though. However, results vary from person to person depending on how committed they are to the process of recovery and the severity of their anxiety disorder. The good news is that anxiety disorders can be treated.

Understanding Your Emotions and Feelings

Emotions and feelings are used interchangeably but are not the same. Emotions are instinctive responses. For example, you see a snake while taking your morning walk and you immediately experience fear. Emotions originate in the limbic part of your brain, which is irrational, illogical, and unreasonable. Emotional reactions may vary slightly between individuals depending on the circumstances but are broadly similar among humans and other species. In other words, other animals such as a dog can understand the emotion behind a smile, for example, and it responds by wagging its tail.

Feelings, on the other hand, are reactions to emotions. They are the mental associations we attribute to our emotions. For example, after seeing the snake during your morning walk, you experience fear and you feel horrified because of what you have heard or previously known about snakes (the mental association).

Emotions play out in your body – you can sense the experience in parts of your body depending on whether you perceive the event as threatening or friendly. Feelings play out in your mind – the arena where events can be interpreted as negative or positive and can also be downplayed or blown out of proportion.

But how does this make any difference in handling anxiety issues? First of all, understanding that your emotions are different from your feelings will help you know what the root cause of your anxiety is. You can then consciously think thoughts and take deliberate actions that are geared toward helping you swim through the murky currents of anxiety. Understanding the difference between your emotions and your feelings will help you live your life from a place of calm response (as Joe did in our earlier example) instead of living from a reactionary place (as Adam did). Your life may not magically transform into a peaceful experience until "happily ever after" because you now know how to respond instead of reacting. But you will be able to find and maintain proper balance irrespective of what is going on around you.

Your emotions are not right or wrong – they are essentially neutral. The way you feel about them, however, could cause you to behave rationally or irrationally. It is okay to experience fear – one of the primary emotions associated with anxiety. But beyond the experience, if you pay attention to what the emotion is telling you, it can guide you to take rational actions. Take your mind back to Adam and Joe trapped in an elevator. Both men perceived the event as threatening, but while Adam reacted to the emotion of fear and behaved irrationally, Joe responded to the same emotion and behaved calmly and rationally. Joe listened to the message of the emotion of fear in his circumstance, "You are trapped. This could be bad." He responded by thinking of how to use the message to his advantage, "How do I get out of this trap?" On the other hand, Adam experienced the emotion of fear, but instead of listening to the message of the emotion, he simply reacted by using learned behaviors from previous experiences. That is behaving on autopilot.

Imagine a woman who endured an abusive relationship for a long time and has had terrible experiences from her spouse before finally getting a divorce. Each time she receives an email from her former partner, she is likely to feel anxious, horrified, and think worrisome thoughts because she has come to associate that feeling with her ex-spouse. Her emotions will automatically make her body react physically (heart pounding, shallow breath, hands shakings, and sweat forming on the face) to a simple email even before she opens it. But if she could begin to gradually take back control of her feelings by being deliberate about her thoughts and behaviors, she would gain control of her automatic reactions. In a nutshell, that is the purpose of this chapter.

How to Avoid Anxious Thoughts

By "avoid," I do not mean ignoring, suppressing, or turning a blind eye to anxious thoughts. You cannot say "I am not going to think this thought" and that thought magically disappears. To begin with, thinking about not thinking a thought is actually thinking that thought (read that again slowly). Also, attempting to monitor your thoughts throughout your waking hours to sift good thoughts from bad ones would impair your day-to-day functions. To successfully avoid anxious thoughts, you have to take the power or the sting out of the thought. Consider it as domesticating a wild animal or castrating a bull – all the bull can do is shoot blanks! When you take out the sting from anxious thoughts, it doesn't matter if the thoughts occur, they will have no power or negative impact on you. Let us discuss how to do just that in three steps: face the thought, create or choose a different thought, and write out the thought and worry about it later.

Face the Thought

The first step to avoid an anxious thought is to face the thought. Turning a blind eye, suppressing it, or avoiding it at all cost is giving more power to the thought. You are subconsciously acknowledging that the fear is too great that you can't face it. But when you confront the thought, you tell it that you are ready to take back control of your thought processes. To face your thoughts, begin to ask yourself whether what you are thinking is helpful or unhelpful. Anxious thoughts are generally irrational and unhelpful. When you question an anxious thought, you will discover that it falls into one of the following categories:

1. **Catastrophic thinking**: A lot of what-ifs characterize this type of thinking. It is focusing on and blowing bad things out of proportion as well as creating unreasonable and imaginary worst-case scenarios. For example, your spouse is not back home on time and you get worried and start thinking they may be involved in an accident or they are dead. This can make you start acting irrationally (like Adam did in the elevator).

Quit tip: When you are beginning to have too many what-ifs running around in your mind, pause and ask yourself: Are my fears based in reality or just my imagination? Realistically, how likely is this to happen? What evidence do I have to confirm these fears?

2. **Overgeneralization**: When you take an isolated event and make it true for everything, you are overgeneralizing. This type of thinking usually focuses on phrases that indicate finality such as "never" and "always." For example, you find out that you are excessively worried about an upcoming event even after you have made up your mind to stop worrying. And then you think, "I'm never going to overcome this worry habit." Or you think, "I'm never going to guess the winning number because I'm always unlucky." The fact is that you are forgetting the saying: never say never. Overgeneralization can make you give up on improvement because you feel you already know the outcome of trying. But the truth is that you are only assuming you know the outcome. Overgeneralization can also make you exaggerate things and become unnecessarily worried. For example, because you failed at something before, you assume that you are going to fail every time you attempt that same thing.

Quick tip: Getting out of the grip of this thought pattern can be achieved by asking yourself: Do I have any concrete evidence to support this line of thinking? Is there something I am not considering here? How do I know that this thing is never this way or always this way?

3. **All-or-nothing thinking**: This is thinking in black or white – it is either this way or no other way! No room for middle ground or gray areas. For example, thinking that if you don't get an A+, you're a total failure. This type of thinking is similar to perfectionism with no room for the complexities of life.

   Quick tip: To break yourself out of this thought pattern, you can begin by asking yourself: How realistic are my expectations? What's the worst that can happen if things are not exactly as I want them to be?

4. **Focusing on the negative**: This is filtering out the positives in your life and dwelling on the negatives. When you allow your mind to ruminate only on the things that are not working well for you, your mind dims the light on your positives and magnifies the negatives. For example, a mother who gives up her day job to take care of her child may become worried about not being able to pacify the child and may begin to think, "*I'm such a bad mother*." But she doesn't acknowledge all the sacrifices she makes for her child. This type of thinking can also make you dismiss the positives in your life as

insignificant or mere flukes. In some cases, it can stop the individual from accepting compliments or praises for performing well.

Quick tip: Getting yourself out of this unhelpful thought can begin by asking yourself: What's the big picture here? Is there something good about this situation I'm ignoring? Can I point out at least one positive thing about this situation?

5. **Jumping to conclusion**: Unless you are a mind reader, you cannot accurately predict what people are thinking. But excessive worrying can make you assume that you know what others are thinking. For example, "She thinks I'm a failure," or "He's not going to accept me." This is mind-reading and predictive thinking. You cannot possibly know for sure what a person is thinking or how they will behave, so it really is a waste of time worrying about it because all it does is to make you jump to a conclusion without concrete evidence.

   Quick tip: To get over this pattern of thinking, ask yourself: What evidence do I have in support of my thinking? Is my evidence based in reality? Would thinking this way help me prepare better for the future or is it exposing me to more worrisome thoughts?

6. **Personalizing**: Thinking that every bad thing that happens around you is your fault is unreasonable. Yet, worrying can make you find irrational connections between you and every type of misfortune. For example, thinking it is your fault that your child failed a test. "I should have allowed him to study hard instead of making him clean up his room." Or your closest friend is in a foul mood and you think, "I must have done something dumb to make her grumpy." Worrying can make you confuse blaming yourself for every misfortune as accepting responsibility for your mistakes.

   Quick tip: Getting over this worrisome thought is a bit tricky, but it can be done if you always remember to ask yourself: How exactly am I responsible for this outcome? Was the situation really under my complete control? Is it rational to blame myself for something I didn't have any control over?

7. **Should, must, and ought**: Standards are good things to live by except that they can become the cages with which we trap ourselves. If your thoughts are always leaning towards what you (or others) should, must, and ought to do, you are setting yourself up for frustration and unnecessary worry. For example, "I should eat only healthy foods", "I must think only positive thoughts," and "I ought to feel better than this." There may be nothing

inherently wrong in wanting to eat healthy food, think positive thoughts, or feel better, but the idea that you should, must, or ought to be doing something or thinking in a certain way can trigger a sense of guilt and blame in you. Instead of setting you on the path of improvement, it can lead to a downward spiral of other negative thoughts. Beating yourself up for not living up to a list of strict rules of what you should and shouldn't do will push you further into anxious thoughts such as, "Now I'm going to gain more weight because I ate what I shouldn't eat."

Quick tip: You can get over this thinking pattern by asking yourself if there are other ways of doing a thing. Challenge "should", "must", and "ought to" thinking by asking what the worst-case scenario would be if you don't follow your rules. You can also question yourself if there is a specific rule that suggests that you must do a thing in a certain way and who made the rule. Realize that everyone makes mistakes and begin to cut yourself some slack whenever you make a mistake.

8. **Emotional reasoning**: The way you feel and the way reality is are two different things but reasoning from an emotional place would not allow you to realize that. Emotional reasoning prevents you from taking actions that can improve yourself or a situation because you feel it won't be worthwhile. For example, "I feel completely

worthless. My boss must be thinking I'm a jerk, and he'll be right." Worrying about how you feel actually hinders you from viewing reality from other perspectives. Emotional reasoning exaggerates your feelings beyond what it really is.

Quick tip: Emotions are a powerful thing, but you can find a way around them by asking: How is this thought helpful to me at this moment? Am I making decisions based on facts or emotions? Can I make sound judgments from an emotional place?

9. **Labeling**: Acting in one particular way does not translate into a habit. But anxiousness has a way of beclouding our judgments and makes us label one act to mean that our entire life is full of that behavior. For example, you couldn't make it to your child's school show and you begin to think, "I am such a disappointment. My whole life is full of broken promises. I am a bad parent." Or you made a mistake in the office that makes your superiors look stupid and then you label yourself as a complete idiot who can't do anything right. That is an extreme generalization, and it can keep you worried about making similar mistakes in the future.

   Quick tip: A good way to get a handle on this pattern of thought is by asking: Is doing something once or a few times qualify it as a habit? Am I labeling a particular behavior or labeling myself as a whole based on this one behavior?

Once you take the bold step of facing an anxious thought and question it, it puts you in a better place to take steps to change your response to the thought. But this should be done using baby steps. You should not start by taking on big fears and worries simply because you have identified them as overgeneralization or some other form of unhelpful thought pattern. Start small. For example, if you worry too much about making mistakes during a public presentation, it is a great start to recognize that the thought about the upcoming public presentation making you nervous. Instead of going headlong into the presentation, start by practicing in front of a few of your close friends or family members. This can help you develop resilience to the anxiety.

Create or Choose a Different Thought

Recognizing that you are having an unhelpful thought is the first step in avoiding anxious thoughts. The next step is to create or choose a different helpful thought. To help you choose a better thought, it is a good idea to have a journal where you write down your unhelpful thoughts. This way, you can discover what your automatic negative thoughts (ANTs) are and then consciously work to replace them. Note that the goal is not to paint everything bright. Your negative thoughts may contain some truth. Be honest about your thoughts and work out a plan to correct whatever lapses you may discover.

Here are some examples of how to choose a different thought using a journal.

Negative Thought	***Type of Negative Thought***	***Replace with a Helpful Thought***
I have a bad feeling about this driving test. My son might have an accident.	Catastrophic thinking	Something can indeed go wrong, but it is also possible that nothing bad will happen during my son's driving test. Most people I know do well during their driving tests.

How could I have failed the last question? I must be dumb.	All-or-nothing thinking	I did well on all the other questions. That certainly counts for something. I will keep striving for excellence instead of perfection.

No one likes me.	Jumping to conclusion	I don't know that for sure. I might just be jumping to a wrong conclusion since I don't have any evidence to support that assumption.

I didn't pass the interview. I can never get any decent job.	Overgeneralization	Some people failed several interviews but later got better jobs. I won't allow this incident to define my entire future.

I ought to have been better at this by now.	Should thinking	We all make mistakes and mistakes show that we are growing. I will get better if I remain consistent.

It is also helpful if you can take note of the following:

1. The situation that is causing your anxiety. Try to note who was with you, what you were doing, what time the

thoughts occur, and where you were.

2. The mood you were in during the situation. Try to also note how you felt during the situation. A one-word description would suffice. For example, did you feel guilty, nervous, irritated, or were you overwhelmed?

All these can help you understand how you ANTs play out and what steps you can take to avoid them.

Write Out the Thought and Worry About It Later

This is one simple but effective trick in avoiding anxious thoughts. It involves setting aside time to worry about the thoughts that are bothering you, which you have earlier written down. Instead of trying (and failing) to stop anxious thoughts, simply postpone the anxious thoughts until a later time. This is one time where procrastination can be a helpful habit! The secret to the effectiveness of this trick is simple: writing down thoughts is a lot more difficult than thinking it on the go. The act of writing down worrisome thoughts significantly removes its power to later affect you negatively when you settle down to think about it. Here's how the process works:

1. **Set aside a period for worrying**: Choose a time and place where you will worry. The duration, time, and place

should be always the same. For example, you can choose to set aside 30 minutes of worry from 5:00 pm to 5:30 pm in the living room daily. Note that the timing should not be too close to your bedtime to avoid having anxious thoughts before you sleep. Religiously keep to this time and worry about anything that bothers you during your worry period. Keep the rest of your free of worrying.

2. **Write down your worries**: Because you have set aside time for worrying does not mean anxious thoughts will not creep up in your head in your worry-free time. When the anxious thoughts occur to you, don't fight them off. Simply write them down in your notepad, phone, or computer and tell yourself that you will bring them up during your worry period so there's no need to worry about them at the moment. Writing out your thoughts requires you to take physical action and think about the thoughts you are writing down. The process of writing is harder than simply letting the thought run its course in your head. Writing down your worry is likely to take the steam out of the anxious thought.

3. **Worry about your list**: It is impractical to stop worry. Worry can serve a good purpose and everyone worries from time to time. It only becomes a problem when it becomes excessive, uncontrollable, and negatively impacts your daily activities. So, if you are trying to avoid

anxious thoughts or recover from an anxiety disorder, don't attempt to stop worrying. Instead, during your designated worry period, bring up all the anxious thoughts you have written down and permit yourself to worry about them. This is a more constructive way to worry about your problems and fears. You'll discover that thinking about your worries this way can help you find a balanced perspective because instead of thinking on autopilot, doing this would mean that you are actually evaluating your worries. For example, during your worry period, instead of having catastrophic thinking such as "I'm never going to ride in an elevator again because I can get trapped and die before someone comes to my rescue!" you can consciously think:

- "Is this line of thinking going to help me overcome my fear of elevators or make me more afraid of elevators?"
- "How many people in real life do I know that have died because they were trapped in an elevator?"
- "What is the probability that every elevator I take would stop working?
- "If an elevator stops working, are there people who get notified immediately or does it remain that way indefinitely?"

If you eventually find that your worries are not that

important any more, drop them off your list and add more or simply reduce the duration of the worry period.

Solvable and Unsolvable Worries

It may sound a bit counterintuitive to set aside time to worry when what you are trying to do is to break the worry habit. But here's the thing: if you take a careful look at the suggestion above about creating a worry period, you'll discover that it is actually another name for problem-solving because it helps you to evaluate your situation, think up plans to handle the situation, and then put the plans to work. Typical worrying, on the other hand, is brooding over a situation without a definite plan of action. If what you worry about eventually happens, worrying doesn't prepare you to deal with them.

This brings up the question, are your worries solvable or unsolvable? Solvable worries are those you can immediately start working on. Unnecessary brooding about uncertainties is not a productive use of your time. As soon as a bothersome thought occurs to you, begin to seek an immediate solution. If you can't handle it at that moment, write it down and process it during your productive worry period. For example, if you are knee-deep in debts and unpaid bills, instead of getting anxious over how your bills are piling up and how you may never get out of debt, consider speaking to your creditors about working out a flexible payment plan. If you have determined that your worries are solvable, by all means, start brainstorming to come up with a comprehensive list of every possible solution you can think of. It doesn't matter if the solutions that occur to you at that moment are perfect or not. Your goal is to look for things that you can control and change, instead of trying to factor in every possible reality that may be out of your control. Consider your options and draw out a plan of action, and then begin to execute the plan. Taking action about your worries will greatly lessen the anxiety you feel about the situation.

If you have determined that your worries are unsolvable, then you have no control over the situation, so simply accept the uncertainty. Worrying about uncertainties doesn't change them. If anything, they prevent you from noticing and enjoying the good things you currently have working in your favor. Instead of worrying about whether you will develop a brain tumor someday, for example, there's simply no way for you to know that and certainly, there isn't any productive action you can take about such worries. If you are having headaches, go see a doctor. If you're not having headaches and there's no sign or symptoms of a tumor in your brain (except for a premonition that something bad will happen to you), it is unnecessary to start worrying about it.

Negative Self-Talk = Self Destruction

I began this chapter by stating that events are neutral, but how we interpret the events will determine how we react or respond to them. In other words, our feelings about something depends on what we think about it. If our thoughts define how we feel, it follows that our dominant thinking habit will determine how we habitually feel. Having the "wrong" thoughts would then mean that our feelings and interpretation about most things will be wrong and our behavioral response too will be wrong. What this implies is that if we must have the correct behavioral response to any situation, we must unlearn the negative way of thinking and replace it with a helpful way of thinking so that our feelings and behaviors will reflect our helpful way of thinking.

One of the ways to effectively change how you think is to change your inner self-talk. The way we talk to ourselves in our minds plays a major role in how we see ourselves and feel about ourselves. If your inner self-talk is dominantly negative, it can lead you down the path of self-destruction. Chronic worriers tend to have a very loud negative critic inside their minds. It constantly reminds them of how stupid they are ("You can't do anything right, you idiot!"), how inadequate they are ("You've never been good at this. Why did you even bother to attempt it?"), and how worthless they are ("You can never amount to anything good, and you know it!"). Of course, negative self-talk can take on several other forms, but the bottom line is that instead of motivating you to take action toward improvement, it drags you down into feeling bad about yourself and your situation. This can often leave you feeling intense anxiety about your ability to perform, realistically appraise a situation, and can even spiral into fear-based thinking, like "I'll probably make a fool of myself if I give a presentation."

Stop Letting Your Past Define You

Negative self-talk usually takes a mistake from your past and blows it into an epic blunder. But beyond exaggerating your past failures, it puts the reminder on autopilot such that each time you encounter a similar situation, the mistake of the past is brought to fore in your mind and you are reminded of how incapable, unfit, and unworthy you are.

Negative self-talk can be very limiting and debilitating. It can stop you dead in your tracks and make you feel worthless because the more you repeat to yourself that you can't do something, the more you believe it even if it was not true. You are also likely to start believing that your efforts are not good enough. Instead of aiming to become better, you aim for perfection and put undue pressure on yourself which can create an intense feeling of anxiety. If you should fail in meeting your perfect standard, your inner critic will not spare you! Operating under such pressure can cause you to worry unnecessarily and get you hung up on getting everything perfect from the outset.

Most people recognize that negative self-talk is unhelpful. But merely understanding that negative self-talk is unhelpful doesn't change anything. You will have to develop the habit of catching yourself in the act of berating yourself for you to break free from that habitual way of talking to yourself.

Halting Negative Self-Talk

1. **Catch yourself in the act**: You cannot stop negative self-talk if you can't notice when you are yapping away at yourself. Learn to become more deliberate about noticing how you feel. When you start to feel bad, it is your cue that your inner conversations are tending towards negativity.

2. **Stop trying too hard to think positively**: Trying too hard to think positive thoughts when you are overwhelmed by negativity is like trying to put a smiley face on an empty fuel gauge indicator; it doesn't solve the problem! You'll simply make matters worse because we all have an internal lie detector that goes off when we are telling ourselves lies. Instead of forcing yourself to think

positive thoughts, reach for neutral thoughts. For example, if you trying to shed some weight, instead of turning your negative thoughts from "I'm never going to find a date with these fat thighs" to "I feel great in my body," try something like, "I can shed some weight if I put my heart to it." You are not pushing against the negative thought with a positive thought. You are simply shifting your focus away from the negative thought to a more helpful direction where you can begin to take action about your situation.

3. **Don't exaggerate your mistakes**: When you think you've made a fool of yourself, stop and ask if you really did so badly. Are you actually going to lose your job because of one critical feedback or was it intended to make you seek improvement? Did everyone think you are a loser in the class or were they more concerned about how to present their own projects? By questioning your version of the story or your initial thoughts, you slow down your inner critic and become kinder to yourself.

4. **Reword your thoughts**: Sometimes, rearranging a few words can make a huge difference in how you perceive yourself. For example, instead of thinking "My life is a mess" because you're having a bad day, you could think something like, "It seems I'm having a difficult day today." You are essentially refusing to label and define

your entire life by a small bad fragment and deliberately describing how you feel instead.

5. **Think from your friend's point of view**: Think about what a good friend would say to you in your situation. If the voice in your head doesn't sound like what a good friend would say, then it probably isn't good advice. Also, don't ever say it to yourself if you wouldn't say it to your good friend. For example, if you won't call your good friend a total loser for flunking a test, don't ever call yourself that for failing at anything.

6. **Give your inner critic a goofy name**: Nicknaming your inner critic is one trick that creates a separation between you and the inner negative voice in your head. The sillier the name, the better because that would not only help you see how ridiculous the critical self-talks are, it also makes you less likely to agree to its nasty suggestions and become less threatened by its harshness. You won't go beating up on yourself if you know that "Debby Downer," "The Perfectionist," "The Gremlin," or "The Nag" is at it again. The more you recognize the inner critic for what it is, the weaker the emotional grip it has on you and eventually, your anxiety cycle is short-circuited.

7. **Realize that negative self-talk is a habit and not necessarily valid feedback**: If you take just a little time to observe your inner narrative, you'll discover that it follows a similar pattern. The feedback is usually the same and consistent around the same theme: you're not good enough, you didn't do well enough, and so on. It is just a habit of thought and not valid feedback. Stop taking it seriously.

8. **Embrace your shortcomings**: Perfectionism is not only going to hurt you, but is it is also a huge burden and a very conducive environment for your inner critic to grow stronger and louder. Stop holding yourself to some incredibly high standards. Cut yourself some slack and get in touch with your human side. Come to terms with the fact that it is okay to mess up and move on – that is the path to genuine improvement and true happiness.

9. **Talk to someone**: Sharing what you are thinking is often a good way to weaken the hold of the inner critic. Your inner critic thrives in secrecy – in the secret recess of your mind. Exposing its rants to a trusted friend can help a lot. For example, if you made a fool of yourself at your in-law's, instead of leaving the place in shame and beating up on yourself, pick up the phone and share your experience and the thoughts in your head with a friend. "I think I just earned the award for stupidity this year!" You

may end up having a good laugh and seeing how ridiculous some of your thoughts can be. In some other cases, talking with someone you trust can also be supportive. Even if you don't talk to someone, just saying the thought out loud can make you see how unrealistic and untrue they are – your cue to give yourself a break.

10. **Use thought-stopping**: This method works for a lot of people. By simply saying the word "Stop!" out loud when you catch yourself saying nasty things like, "I'm never going to get this right," "I'm a total failure," or "I'm such a dumb fool!" Other ways to use thought-stopping could be just visualizing a stop sign, snapping your finger, pinching yourself, or snapping a rubber band on your wrist – just anything to snap you out of the negative thought. The next step after halting the negative self-talk is to replace it with something more helpful. For example, when you catch yourself thinking, "I'm going to make a fool of myself," say out loud, "Stop!" And then say something like, "I've been in situations that made me very anxious before, but somehow I succeeded. This situation is no different. I can do this!" Sometimes, it takes more than one stop command or snapping action to get you out of the clutches of the negative self-talk. But if you continue to use the stop command or cue and repeat your helpful thought, you will eventually gain mastery

over the negative chatter.

Chapter 3: Exercises for Managing Anxiety

An anxious mind is a mind that is not at rest. To effectively manage such minds, efforts must be geared toward quieting down the restlessness. This chapter is focused on exposing you to a couple of exercises that can help to put you in a state of calmness and peace – to calm your mind from the activities that cause anxiety. But before we go into the exercises, let us take a brief look at the sympathetic and parasympathetic nervous systems to help us understand how our bodies respond instinctively to stimuli, how our body functions are controlled and regulated, and how we can take advantage of this knowledge to manage excessive anxiety and worry.

Sympathetic Nervous System vs. Parasympathetic Nervous System

The autonomic nervous system is part of the nervous system that is responsible for involuntary regulating the internal functions of our body. It is further divided into the sympathetic nervous system (SNS) and the parasympathetic nervous system (PNS). Both of these systems work involuntarily – that is, without our conscious control – to regulate a group of bodily functions. However, their work is exactly opposite to each other.

The SNS is in charge of what is commonly known as the fight-or-flight response. On the other hand, the PNS is responsible for the rest-and-digest response. Let me paint a little scenario to help us get a clear picture of how these two systems work.

Imagine for a minute that you are in the savannah all by yourself and enjoying the soothing sounds and the great views when all of a sudden you see an angry-looking tiger walking into your path. In that instant, your brain recognized the tiger as a threat and immediately, the SNS kicks in without any effort on your part. Within seconds, the following takes place inside your body:

- Your pupils are dilated to show surprise or shock.

- Your heart rate is increased to supply nutrients and oxygen to your muscles and brain to help you prepare to deal with the situation (either to fight or run).

- Glucose is released into your bloodstream by your liver to boost your energy level and power your muscles just in case you have to use them.

- Dilation takes place in your lungs to help you get more air into the lungs. You need more air to keep up with the increased flow of blood because of the increased heart rate.

- Your adrenal glands secrete hormones to make you more alert and reinforce the effect of the fight-or-flight response of the SNS.
- All digestive activities are put on hold to enable you to muster every ounce of energy in your body.

Other bodily functions are involuntarily regulated in such situations, but this covers some of the major functions. Suppose you chose to run for dear life instead of fighting the tiger (which is a very sane option!) and ran as far and as quickly as you can. When you eventually stop running because you're no longer in danger of being devoured, your PNS kicks into action. It begins the exact opposite of what the SNS has done by relaxing your body to make it recover from the heightened state of metabolic and physical activity. The PNS begins to:

- Decrease your heart rate.
- Relax your muscles.
- Constrict your pupils.
- Returns your digestive functions and your body to a state of calm.

So, how does this relate to managing your anxiety? We live in a time where we are not often exposed to life-threatening dangers such as encountering an angry-looking tiger. However, we are exposed to situations that make us respond as if we are faced with life-threatening danger. For many people, the very second they open their eyes in the morning, thoughts of unpaid bills, overdue rent, poor sanitary condition, relationship issues, sick kids, commuting to a job they hate, pressure at work, poor health, poor body image, low self-esteem, and a host of other problems get their SNS on overdrive! Your body is meant to be in a relaxed state most of the time. It should only be geared up for action when faced with danger. But modern life seems to have flipped the coin, making the agitated state the default state for many people. Chronic worrying can put the body in a constant fight-or-flight mode, which can eventually affect the physical and psychological health of the individual.

> "Over time, repeated activation of the stress response takes a toll on the body. Research suggests that chronic stress contributes to high blood pressure, promotes the formation of artery-clogging deposits, and causes brain changes that may contribute to anxiety, depression, and addiction" (Harvard Health Publishing, 2011).

In simple English, if your survival mechanism (fight-or-flight response) is always activated, it impairs your physical and psychological health. This is why chronic worriers develop anxiety disorders. Instinctively, we know that a state of anxiety – a heightened state of physical and metabolic activity – isn't a good place to be. In a bid to get ourselves back to a normal relaxed state, some people resort to substances, such as alcohol and drugs, to put them in a calm and relaxed state. Unfortunately, this is also not a healthy option. The best option is to stimulate your PNS to help your body and mind relax naturally.

Some of the negative impacts of remaining in a continuous state of fight-or-flight mode include:

- Hardening the arteries, high blood pressure, and heart attack.
- Diarrhea or chronic constipation.
- Sexual impotence, decreased energy levels, type 2 diabetes, and decreased longevity.
- Decreased rate of muscle recovery after training.

On the other hand, the benefits of spending most of your time in a relaxed state include:

- Lower blood pressure, higher heart rate variability, and lower risk of a heart attack.

- Less risk of developing diabetes.
- Increased energy levels due to a balanced level of cortisol.
- Better and improved sleep quality.

The rest of this chapter is focused on ways in which you can stimulate your PNS to significantly reduce worrisome and intrusive thoughts and decrease the physical and psychological impacts of anxiety. Note that you should not engage in any of these exercises when driving or operating machinery.

Mindfulness Exercises

Mindfulness is deliberately bringing your awareness to the present moment. It involves taking a moment to really hear the sounds, perceive the smells, see the sights, taste the food and drinks, and to feel your environment. It also means taking some time to think calmly about the thoughts and emotions you feel without judgment, evaluation, or thinking in terms of right or wrong.

In a world where multitasking seems to be the order of the day, slowing down and becoming fully involved and aware of one after the other seems out of place. But it is the act of being in a hurry – trying to do so many things at the same time – that puts us under undue pressure and activates our SNS. Mindfulness stimulates the PNS and keeps the body in a relaxed state for an extended period.

Benefits of Mindfulness

Some of the health benefits of mindfulness include:

- Reduce dependency on opioid drugs (Science Daily, 2014).
- Reduce the pain associated with arthritis and asthma (Medical Daily, 2013).
- Improve sleep quality especially in older adults (Black et al, 2015).
- Improve heart rate (International Journal of Behavioral Medicine, 2015).
- Healthier glucose levels, improved focus, lower anxiety and depression levels, relieve physical stress, and prevent health issues (Medical Daily, 2016).
- Beneficial effects on the DNA of breast cancer patients (Carlson et al, 2014).

Generally, a person with anxiety has difficulty dealing with intrusive and distracting thoughts especially when the thoughts are repetitive and bothersome. The difficulty arises because the person can't seem to distinguish between a nagging thought that is not beneficial and a problem-solving thought. They might be running late for work and then think, "I'm very late. If I don't get to work on time, I might lose my job! I am such a disorganized person!" The practice of mindfulness helps the person to recognize and acknowledge the thought in a nonjudgmental way and leave it for what it is without attributing meaning to it. For example, a person running late could simply observe, "That's the anxious thought again. It is just a thought and nothing more. It doesn't define me."

Suggested Mindfulness Exercises

I recommend practicing the following mindfulness exercises several times a day for short periods (5 minutes is great). There's no need to stretch your mindfulness practice for an entire hour at a time; doing that is worrying about getting rid of worry!

1. **Getting in Touch with Your Senses and Surroundings**

    - As you go about your daily activities become more deliberate about the actions you take and how you feel about those activities instead of performing your actions on autopilot. For example, when walking, try and notice how your body feels during the walk. Don't zone out. Take note of the scenery and your surroundings as you walk. When you open a door, for example, touch the handle and feel how the handle feels in your hand. Try to ask yourself how things feel.

- Listen to sounds around you – in your office or cubicle, at home, or on the street. What smells do you perceive? What does your food or drink taste like? Your focus should be on simply observing your senses to get a feel of them.
- Whether you are on the beach or in your garden, stand barefoot and feel the sand beneath your feet. Notice the air blowing against your skin and just take it in for a moment.

2. **Mindful Eating**

- When you are eating, concentrate on the food and really enjoy it. Turn off the television, put your cell phone away, and shut down your laptop or computer. Don't allow technology to rob you of the enjoyment that comes from eating.
- Deliberately chew your food and savor every bite. You will enjoy the taste better and feel more satisfied. This will likely result in less temptation to snack afterward.

- Be deliberate about chewing your food. You can close your eyes for a few seconds to allow you to focus on all the tastes and deliciousness of your food.

3. **Slowing Down**

- Handle your tasks one at a time. There is really no need to multitask. When one task is completed, take a quick break to notice your environment and relish in your moments before beginning another task. Your mind and body will thank you for keeping stress out of your daily tasks be performing them this way.
- If there is no emergency, practice letting things occur naturally without giving in to the urge to intercept things. Unless it is very necessary, try to let things play out.

4. **Changing Your Routine**

- A lot of the times we miss out on the efforts required to perform a task because we have performed them so many times we can now do them effortlessly. Try to change how you do things and you will become more aware of the effort required to accomplish the task and also become more aware of the task you are performing. For example, use your non-dominant hand to comb your hair, write, or do the dishes.

- Changing your routine can also make you more alert. If you want to get tuned in with your tasks, change how you do them, and you'll perform those effortless tasks more consciously.

5. Noticing Your Thoughts

- Go to a place where you will not be disturbed for about 5 to 15 minutes. Sit quietly in a comfortable position and observe your thoughts. Do not resist, control, or try to stop your thoughts. Simply let them occur naturally and notice them as if you are an outside observer.
- If you can, label your thoughts as they occur. Don't categorize them as good or bad and don't evaluate them as appropriate or inappropriate. Simply name them. For example, a thought crosses your mind and says, "I'm getting too fat! My partner is not going to find me attractive anymore." Notice it and name it out loud or silently, "That's a thought about not being good enough." Or your thoughts may go something like, "If everything works out as planned, I should be debt-free by next month." Notice it and name it, "That's an optimistic thought."
- Continue to notice and name your thoughts this way for the duration of this exercise. You are essentially allowing yourself to become aware of your thought

processes. Over time, you will be able to deliberately shift your focus to thoughts and actions that are beneficial to you.

Mindfulness is about learning to accept your world from a perspective of curious observation. When you get the hang of it, you will discover that you are more accepting of your worrisome thoughts instead of reacting and letting them upset you. Over time, worry and anxiety are likely to gradually diminish and lose their power over you.

Meditation Exercises

People use meditation and mindfulness interchangeably, but they are a bit different. While it is not the focus of this book to go into the esoteric meanings or uses of any of these practices, it is important to clarify the difference between these two. In simple terms, mindfulness (as can be seen in the previous section) is being aware of "something" (where something could be any activity), and meditation is being aware of "nothing" – essentially clearing away as many thoughts as possible. In a way, mindfulness is a form of meditation. Different forms of meditations have been developed over the years to suit different religions and cultures. However, we shall only concern ourselves with how it can be used to reduce stress and improve the quality of our thoughts.

Typically, to meditate, a person sits and focuses their attention inward to increase concentration, emotional balance, and calmness. Depending on the type of meditation, a person could focus on their breath, chant a certain word or phrase known as a mantra, visualize certain good-feeling imagery, or listen to some recorded sounds or instructions known as guided meditation. During meditation, you spend a focused chunk of time in deliberating concentration while minimizing distractions.

Suggested Meditation Practice to Decrease Anxiety

Here's a meditation exercise I'll suggest you try to help calm you down and stimulate your PNS. Don't worry, we are not going into any form of spiritual or esoteric practice. The focus here is to reduce anxiety. Remember to set a timer to a time that is comfortable for you. You don't have to begin with a full hour of meditation. I recommend you begin with 5 minutes and gradually increase the time as you get better at it. Remember to take baby steps. Also, I strongly suggest that you make the practice a daily one. This meditation helps to bring your focus to your breath and nothing more.

1. Sit upright in a comfortable chair and in a location where

you will not be disturbed or distracted throughout your meditation. It is advisable to turn off your cell phone, put it on silent, or put it far away from you (unless you need to use it to set your timer).

2. Close your eyes and take some time (about a minute) to take in a few deep breaths to get you settled.

3. Now breathe normally and pay attention to how the breath goes in and out.

4. Things may happen within and around you that can shift your focus, but gently bring your focus back to your breath as it goes in and out.

5. When anxious or worrisome thoughts cross your mind, don't fight them. Simply acknowledge them and bring your focus back to your breathing.

6. Remain in this nonjudgmental observation for the duration of your meditation.

7. When your timer goes off, take a few moments to remain quietly seated before opening your eyes.

8. Notice how you feel without evaluation. Simply observe how you feel.

When you first start this practice, it is likely to feel very weird. I mean, how can sitting still and thinking of nothing get you out of all the pressing problems you have? What do you possibly stand to gain with this practice? Well, the practice may not immediately get you out of your pressing problems and you may not gain anything, but you certainly will lose a lot of things such as insecurity, anxiety, pent-up anger, depression, and fear of death.

What If You Just Can't Practice Meditation?

Some people find it extremely difficult to just sit around breathing when there's a lot that needs to be done. Others have trouble observing without being judgmental and even when they try to relax, so many negative thoughts keep running around in their heads. And for some, the thought of doing absolutely nothing except to relax is simply unthinkable. If you find it difficult to practice meditation, you need to keep the following in mind:

- You need to give yourself time. Your first few meditation sessions may not be without obstacles but that should be expected. You've spent your entire life being action-oriented, it is normal to have a difficult time learning to not do anything. It takes practice to learn how to get things done; it also takes practice to learn how to do nothing. So, stick with the practice. You will get better with time.

- Use a mantra. If your thoughts keep wondering and you're finding it frustrating, you can introduce a mantra to help you focus on "nothing." A one or two-syllable word is okay as a mantra. You can use any word as long as it doesn't cause more distractions or cause your mind to wander off on all tangents. This is why people who use mantras stick to "meaningless" or non-thought-provoking chants such as "ohm" to help them improve their focus on their breath during meditations. If this sounds too religious for your liking, you can ignore it completely.
- You also need to make time for the practice of meditation. Don't skip it or make it optional. Always make time for it no matter how busy your schedule is. It can help you to become more centered to handle whatever is thrown at you during your day.

Breathing Exercises

"But wait! Is this actually necessary? I have been breathing for like ages and I'm still worried sick about everything! How does breathing change anything?"

It's not surprising to get reactions like the above from people who don't understand the efficacy behind deliberate breathing. You can drive from work back to your house without consciously being aware of all the movements of your hands and feet while driving your car. In that case, your hands and feet were on autopilot. That is how a lot of people breathe all of their lives – on autopilot. Therefore, they do not consciously tap into the immense benefits of deliberate breathing.

To know how to use breathing to ease anxiety, you need to first understand that there are two types of breathing patterns, namely:

1. **Chest or thoracic breathing**: This is taking shallow breaths from the chest. Usually, it happens unconsciously when people become anxious. The breaths are rapid and stimulate the SNS. Breathing from the chest, which a lot of people are used to, is a poor breathing habit. "Overly rapid breathing can induce feelings of stress and anxiety. This phenomenon is used in behavioral therapy sessions to train anxious patients to confront their emotions directly. By deliberately hyperventilating, patients artificially trigger an unpleasant anxiety, which they get accustomed to feeling and learn to put in perspective. This technique also enables them to see that poor breathing habits amplify their fear" (Andre, 2019).

2. **Abdominal or diaphragmatic breathing**: These are deep and even breaths. This is usually the breathing pattern when you reach the relaxed stage during your sleep. Healthy newborns also breathe this way. While it may not be practical for many people to breath this way all of the time, it is important to observe how you breathe, especially when you are under stress or anxious, and do your best to breath from your abdomen.

Suggested Breathing Exercise for Relaxation

The following are some breathing exercises you can try when next you feel anxious. Repeat any of these for up to three times a day for about 5 to 10 minutes to give you relief from sporadic stress. If you make this a habit by doing it daily, you will likely experience lower levels of anxiety in your day-to-day activities. Whether you are standing, sitting, or lying down when you do the breathing exercise, remember to maintain a straight posture – shoulders back, no stiffness, just relaxing.

1. **Abdomen Breathing**

   This technique can help you master breathing from the diaphragm and stimulate the PNS while at the same time help in reducing the amount of work done by your body to breathe properly.

- Sit or lie down comfortably.
- Place one hand just above your belly button and the other on your chest.
- Gently inhale through your nose so that the air goes down into your stomach. If you are doing this correctly, you'll notice that there's almost no movement in your chest. If your chest is rising and falling (you'll know by observing the hand on your chest), try isolating your breathing so that your stomach rises and falls instead.
- Gently breathe out through your pursed lips. Contract your stomach muscles to push the air out as you exhale.
- Continue for the next 5 to 10 minutes.

You may notice that it is a bit tiring to breathe this way if this is the first time you are doing this. But it will get easier over time, and you'll be glad you persisted in practicing it.

2. **Breath Focus**

This technique helps you to take deep slow breaths in and out while focusing on calming words.

- Breathe normally and notice how it feels when you inhale and exhale. Perform a mental scan of your body while breathing normally to notice if you feel any form of tension.

- Now take a deep slow breath through your nose. Notice how your upper body and belly expand.
- Breathe out in whichever way you choose.
- Repeat this for several minutes while paying attention to how your belly rises and falls.
- Choose a calming word to focus on and repeat silently and you breathe out. Use words like peace, calm, or safe.
- When you breathe in, imagine the inhale as a gentle wave washing over you.
- When you breathe out, imagine the exhale sweeping away your upsetting and worrisome thoughts out of your body.
- If you get distracted, gently return your attention to your chosen word and you breathe in and out.
- Continue for the next 10 minutes or more if you have the time.

3. **Equal Breathing**

This technique ensures that your inhale and exhale occur for the same amount of time.

- Close your eyes. Breathe several times and notice your normal breath.

- Now slowly count 1, 2, 3, and 4 while inhaling through your nose.
- Repeat the same slow count while exhaling.
- Notice how the air fills and empties from your lungs as inhale and exhale.
- Your counting pace may vary as you continue breathing and counting. It is okay as long as you keep the counts for inhaling and exhaling the same.

4. **Resonant Breathing**

This is similar to the Equal Breathing technique but with longer counts, and it is recommended to be done while lying down to help you get into a more relaxed state.

- For this exercise, lie down on your back and close your eyes.
- With your mouth closed, gently inhale through your nose for 6 seconds. Let the air fill your lungs gradually but don't fill it with too much air.
- Now exhale for another 6 seconds. Don't rush the exhale. Let the air flow out gradually and gently.
- Continue for about 10 minutes.
- When you have completed this exercise, remain lying down and pay attention to how your body feels.

5. **Longer Exhale**

   Inhaling deeply may not calm you down especially when done rapidly. Instead, it can stimulate the SNS and can even cause you to hyperventilate. This method of breathing tilts the scale in favor of exhaling for longer periods. This can help in stimulating the PNS.

   - Stand, sit, or lie down.
   - Instead of beginning with a deep breath in, begin by exhaling thoroughly. Consciously empty the air from your lungs.
   - Now allow your lungs to inhale air without forcing it.
   - As you breathe this way, make sure that you exhale for a little bit longer than you inhale. For example, you can exhale for 6 seconds and then breathe in for 4 seconds.
   - Continue to do this for about 2 to 5 minutes.

Whichever technique of breathing you choose to use, it is helpful if you think reassuring thoughts during the exercise. For example, when you inhale, think thoughts such as "I breathe in tranquility" and when you exhale, think "I breathe out stress."

Exercise Therapy

Physical exercise has several physical benefits among which are improved sleep, increased sexual interest, improved mood, increased stamina and energy levels, weight reduction, improved cardiovascular fitness, among others (Sharma, et al, 2006). It is also considered vital for stress reduction and "a viable treatment option for the treatment of anxiety" (Aylett, Small, and Bower, 2018).

To be clear, physical exercise will not cure your anxiety disorder, but the psychological and physical benefits of exercise can significantly improve the symptoms of anxiety. While any good exercise can help to reduce anxiety, aerobic exercises, those that can really get your heart pumping, are more beneficial. Some of these include swimming, dancing, brisk walking, running, biking, and tennis. Performing any of these activities between 15 to 30 minutes for about 3 to 5 days a week can greatly improve symptoms.

Yoga

Yoga is Sanskrit for "unite." The practice "unites" the body and mind using a combination of different postures that stretches and strengthens your core while you take focused breaths. This combination significantly slows down your mind and creates a sense of personal balance and tranquility in you. Anxiety, as we have seen in a previous chapter, has physical symptoms such as tightness, feelings of tension, and pain sensitivity. Yoga postures can relief the physical discomfort associated with anxiety (Star, 2019).

The following are some suggested yoga poses to help you calm your anxious mind. It is recommended to spend about 3 to 5 minutes doing a pose before switching to a different one.

1. **Cat/Cow Pose**

   As you perform this pose, keep your eyes closed to help you pay attention to the movements and your breath.

   - Go down on your hands and feet. Keep your back straight, knees directly under your hip bone, and your hands straight under your shoulders.
   - Take in a deep breath and lower your belly so that your back is arched. Pull your shoulder blades in as you expand your chest and lift your gaze. This is the Cow Pose.
   - Let the air out as you push down on your palms, curve your back, and bring your gaze down toward your navel. This is the Cat Pose.
   - Repeat these poses as you inhale and exhale and let your breath find a rhythm with each movement.
   - Slowly switch from one pose to the other so that you can feel the movement in your spine.

2. **Standing Forward Bend**

You don't need a mat for this pose and it can be done anywhere.

- Stand with your feet slightly apart or together.
- Raise your arms above your head, keeping your spine straight. Bend forward and let your arms hold your elbows as your head hangs down toward your toes.
- Feel as the tension is gradually released from your head, shoulders, and upper back.
- Let your eyes close softly as you take slow deep breaths in and out.
- Release any thought and maintain the pose for as long as is comfortable.

3. **Legs Up the Wall**

- Place your mat very close to a wall that can support your legs when you stretch them.
- Curl up on your side and then move your hips so that it is against the wall. Turn on your back and stretch your legs to rest upright against the wall.
- If you feel any tension in your lower back with your leg up against the wall, put a pillow under your hips.
- Let your arms rest gently by your side. Open your palms and let them face up.

- Now close your eyes and pay attention to your breath.
- Inhale deeply for a count of five and repeat the same on the exhale.
- Stay in this position for as long as you can while you let go of all tension. Your heart rate will slow down as you hold this pose.

4. **Corpse Pose**

- Lie flat on your back on top of your mat. Let your arms rest loosely by your side with your palms facing up. Relax your legs so that your feet point to the sides of your mat.
- If you feel any tension in your lower back, place a pillow under the back of your knees for support.
- Gently let your eyes close and let go of any tension you may feel in your face.
- Begin to inhale and exhale deeply until you feel very relaxed.

5. **Child's Pose**

- Kneel on a thick mat or folded blanket. You can spread your knees or keep them together. Make sure that the mat or folded blanket is thick enough to make your knees comfortable.
- Raise both arms up and then stretch them in front of

you.

- Gently close your eyes.
- Release any tension you feel in your head, neck, shoulders, arms, back, and let go of intrusive thoughts as you bring your arms down on the mat, stretching them as far in front of you as you can.
- Let your body rest on your thighs. Soften any tension you feel in your muscles. As you breathe in and out, allow yourself to relax deeply. Find peace and tranquility in this pose.

Ways to Find Instant Calm

Victor Frankl once said, “Between stimulus and response, there is a space. In that space is our power to choose our response. In our response lies our growth and our freedom.” Many times, we feel as if we are at the mercy of stressful events – as if we have no control over the things that happen to us. At such times, our minds become filled with scary stories and images about possible unwanted outcomes, whose fault is it that we are in such situations, or how inadequate we are for being in such situations. But these are not necessarily true because we actually do have a lot of control. We can take creative control over almost any situation. Taking control doesn't necessarily mean instantly changing the situation. But it means responding differently to the situation. In this section, we shall take a look at how to instantly regain control of upsetting situations to bring about instant calm.

Positive Self-Talk

When you repeat something frequently enough, your mind believes it regardless of whether it is true. The effect of repeating positive words or affirmations to yourself is like the effect of a gentle but constant stream of water on a rock – it will wear the rock down! Unfortunately, the same is true for repeating negative words to yourself.

For this technique to be effective, I strongly suggest that you make positive self-talk your default way of thinking and talking about yourself. Do not wait until you are in a stressful situation before you practice positive self-talk. It is likely to backfire because your internal lie detector is always active and knows when you are lying to yourself. Your mind is a more fertile ground to receive positive self-talk when you are not exposed to stressors. If you take the time to predominantly fill your mind with positive self-talk, stressful situations will only activate the positivity in you to counterbalance the negative stressor. However, the opposite is true if your mind is filled with negative self-talk.

Here are some suggested affirmations or positive phrases you can constantly repeat to yourself. Keep in mind that your choice of positive words should be personal and meaningful to you.

1. I am lovable.
2. I am capable.
3. Most people I encounter are lovable and capable too.
4. I am calm, cool, and collected.
5. A challenge is my opportunity for growth.
6. I can make changes and I can cope with changes.
7. It is human to make mistakes, and they are a sign that I am taking action.
8. My world is full of great things.
9. My life is wonderful.
10. Everything is working out for me.

In some situations, you may find yourself in a very negative frame of mind that the thought of bringing yourself to think or say anything positive infuriates you the more. Let it play out. Don't force positive self-talks in such situations. Instead, try to soften the negativity by using milder words. Notice how nurses would rather say "discomfort" instead of "pain." That's an example of mild wording and it has a significant impact on the mind. Instead of using strong saying things like, "I hate waiting" or "I am so angry," consider softer words like "I don't like waiting" or "I am so annoyed." You are essentially saying the same thing but more mildly and your body will also respond mildly instead of being so tensed up.

Guided Imagery

Guided imagery, like creative visualization, is the act of deliberately distracting oneself from the cause of stress or worry to an alternative focus, which usually involves evoking a mentally peaceful environment. Creative visualization involves using all your senses to picture yourself in a setting as if it were on a mental screen. This could be visualizing yourself with better health, relationships, jobs, or whatever it is you would like to change in your life. You are seeing the result in your mind. But with guided imagery, you or someone else is guiding you through a series of visualizations. That is to say, there is a plot or storyline – a beginning, middle, and an end – to the visualization. For example, if you are using guided imagery to help you eliminate worry, you may begin by picturing yourself in the beautiful scenery and seeing a bright light flowing into your body as you inhale, exploding as it collides with your source of worry, and then flowing out of your body as you exhale.

If you get a massage or have some other physical relaxation technique while practicing guided imagery, your mind associates the comfortable feelings and sensations you get from the relaxation with the peaceful images in your mind. This means that your mind will activate the sensations each time you begin your guided imagery sessions.

This is a rather easier technique to use compared to yoga or other forms of exercise, especially if you have some type of physical limitation. However, the technique takes some practice to truly activate your mental guide, unlike the breathing exercises where all you need is to focus on your breath.

There is no one correct way to use guided imagery to relieve stress. Here is a general guide.

1. Go to a place where you will not be disturbed and make yourself comfortable.
2. Breathe slowly and deeply for a few moments to help you become calmer.
3. Now softly close your eyes.
4. Picture yourself in a beautiful setting. It could be in your favorite room, in a forest, on a mountain, by the beach, and so on. Just imagine that everything is ideal in your environment.
5. Imagine that you are having a good time being happy, relaxed, or calm.
6. Etch on your mind the different attributes of your scene by focusing on them more vividly. For example, if you choose to picture yourself by the beach, notice the sand under your feet, the gentle breeze and warmth of the sun on your skin, the sound of the waves, the smell of the

ocean, and so on. Engage as many of your physical senses as you can to help you make the image clearer in your mind.

7. Remain in that state of imagination for about 5 to 10 minutes.
8. When you are feeling relaxed, tell yourself that you can come back to this special location anytime you choose to.
9. Gently open your eyes and return to your daily activity.

Tips

- You can use ambient sounds that are compatible with your imagery to obscure real-life sounds while using this stress relief technique.

- You may want to consider using audio recordings from a therapist or even visiting a therapist to guide you during your sessions. If you prefer the sound of your voice, you could also play a record of your voice to guide you during the session.

- Remember to set an alarm so that your mind won't get distracted by your waiting schedule. Also, in the event that you fall asleep, an alarm will wake you up.

Practice Gratitude

Gratitude goes beyond just saying thank you. It is not being grateful about everything because that would be ridiculous – you certainly shouldn't be grateful for having anxiety! Gratitude is not a magic wand that makes anxiety go away in a poof! However, it can rewire your brain and provide the following scientifically proven benefits (Psychology Today, 2015):

- Gratitude releases toxic emotions from your mind.
- Gratitude reduces pain.
- Gratitude improves sleep quality.
- Gratitude reduces anxiety and depression.
- Gratitude aids in stress regulation (National Institute of Health, 2017).

Here are some ways you can practice gratitude to help you manage anxiety.

1. **Get a gratitude pal**: Sometimes, getting one or two like-minded people to work with you creates a multiplier effect on what you are working on. Find someone or a few people who would like to practice the act of gratitude with you and spend a few minutes every day to discuss what

you are truly grateful for. Your gratitude pal could be your friend, your child, or your spouse. Your discussions should be informal and open, and questions should be welcomed.

2. **Keep a gratitude journal**: A gratitude journal is like your diary, but you record only things that you are thankful for in it whether they are small or big things. As you record what you are grateful for, deliberately choose to focus on the pleasant emotions and good memories associated with the events you are writing down. Your gratitude journal can follow this pattern.

Gratitude Journal	
Things I like about myself.	1.
	2.
	3.
	4.

People I am grateful for.	1.
	2.
	3.
	4.
Things that are working well for me.	1.
	2.
	3.
	4.
What I am learning from my current challenges.	1.
	2.

	3.
	4.

3. **Appreciate yourself**: Take a good look at yourself in a mirror and say five good things about yourself. Speak them out aloud. It doesn't matter whether they are in the past or present, just appreciate yourself out aloud. Use positive words such as loving, kind, multitalented, disciplined, loyal, and so on to describe yourself. If you can't find anything pleasant to say about yourself in the moment, simply stare at your reflection in the mirror and smile. Keep smiling until you feel a shift in how you feel then begin to appreciate yourself. Repeat this practice as often as possible and observe how you feel afterward.

4. **Make a list**: This is similar to keeping a gratitude journal but without going into the minute details. In simple terms, this is what "count your blessings" means. Take a sheet of paper or open a new page on your computer or mobile device and write out a list of all the

people who offered you support in one form or the other and write what they did for you. Try to get into the state you were when the actual event occurred. When you are done writing, go over it for about 2 minutes and feel truly grateful before putting the list away. Your list should look like this:

Gratitude List	
I am grateful to...	For...
1.	
2.	
3.	
4.	
5.	

5. **Gratitude notes**: Follow your gratitude list with a thank

you note to as many people as you can remember. Freely express your gratitude in the notes you send to the people on your gratitude list without expecting any response from them. You could send the notes as emails, text messages, or even handwrite them.

Touching Your Lips

Have you ever wondered why when you put a finger on your lips, almost anyone will recognize it as a sign to be quiet? Whatever the reason for that is is not as important as the effect that simple gesture produces both on others and on your mind and body. It doesn't just quiet others; it can also quiet the mind from unnecessary worries and fears by stimulating the PNS.

Your lips have parasympathetic nerve fibers spread across them. So when you lightly run a finger or two over your lips, it stimulates the PNS. According to Rick Hanson, Ph.D., here are some reasons why this method works (Hanson, 2007):

- Fiddling the lips stimulates the PNS nerve fibers spread throughout the lips. This sends reverberations in the entire PNS.

- Touching the lips can trigger the good-feeling emotions associated with thumb-sucking, feeding, and nursing.

- Lightly touching the lips can stimulate salivation. People don't usually salivate in the face of danger, when they are worried and anxious, or when their fight-or-flight response is activated. Salivation is a function majorly controlled by the PNS – the rest-and-digest response.

- The simple act of touching your lips can also distract you from whatever is bothering you because of its sheer absurdity.

Creativity and Hobbies

Sometimes, practices that tend toward esoteric concepts may seem inadequate to deal with our anxiety. Some people would prefer something more practical or hands-on to give them a sense of doing. This is not surprising considering that we live in an action-oriented world. If you find it difficult to get your mind away from worrisome thoughts through some of the other techniques described above, perhaps you could try focusing on doing something creative. Keep in mind that when you are trying to use creative activity to distract your mind from worries, the activities should be performed for fun. You don't want to add the stress of seriousness to your list of worries. Develop a hobby that you can turn to every once in a while to clear your mind of anxious thoughts. Some of the hobbies or creative activities that you can perform to relieve stress include:

1. Gardening – Exposes you to fresh air and sunshine, and it is a way to create a beautiful environment for yourself.
2. Photography – Gives you a different view of the world around you, gradually shifting your focus from worries to the beauties hidden in plain view.
3. Scrapbooking – Helps you create memories by combining pictures and journaling while giving you a break from stressful concerns.
4. Maintaining an aquarium – Gives you a sense of creating a small world of beautiful aquatic creatures, plant life, and rocks. Regular (but not overwhelming) attention is required to maintain an aquarium – a welcome distraction from worries.
5. Solving puzzles – Can help you improve your brain power aside from distracting you from your worries. Whether it is a crossword or jigsaw puzzle, it can make you experience flow, which can strengthen your ability to think clearly and approach your problems with a fresher and stronger mind.
6. Drawing and painting – Can be a welcome distraction to help you express or process your emotions.
7. Knitting – Provides you an opportunity to engage in a repetitive motion that can put you in a mental state where you experience flow.
8. Playing the piano – Helps fully absorb your attention to express very creative music.

Chapter 4: Managing Your Time, Energy, and Activities

Apart from traumatic experiences and heredity, the constant rush and pressure to get things done is a major contributing factor to anxiety. Having to handle the demands of kids and spouses, work pressure, societal expectations, health and fitness issues, and so on can take its toll on you and lead to worry and anxiety. It is important to learn how to manage your time, energy, and how to prioritize your activities to reduce your chances of developing an anxiety disorder. This chapter briefly discusses how you can effectively plan your daily activities to make you more efficient and, in turn, diminish your anxieties.

Fretting About Time Management vs. Designing Your Day

Each of us has an equal amount of time per day, but while some of us get more things done in the same number of hours, some others spend a large chunk of their time fretting about how to manage their time. Many people do not really understand the difference between lack of time, energy management skills, and time management skills. First of all, there is no such thing as a lack of time. You cannot increase, reduce, steal, beg, or borrow extra time; it is fixed. You are either using it well or not. When you think that you are running a race against time, you inadvertently set yourself up for constant worry because you will never win the race against time; no one ever has and no one ever will. That leaves you with developing your time management skills as well as your energy management skills.

If you understand when your productive energy is at its peak and you design your important activities around that time, you are using both time and energy efficiently. But if you merely schedule your activities without regard to your energy levels, you may be attempting to manage your time well but ignoring your ability to handle stress.

Go ahead and ask yourself what you enjoy doing the most, what times of the day you tend to be more active, and what things are most important to you, and then deliberately design your activities to fit into your peak periods.

Prune Your Daily To-Do List

We often think time management means creating a to-do list. Having what you want to be done written down can give you a sense of direction and accomplishment but only if you accomplish the tasks written down. If you don't complete your tasks, your to-do list can become a source of anxiety. At the end of the day, when you take a look at your long list of uncompleted tasks, you begin to feel like a total failure and a loser! Instead of giving you a sense of accomplishment, it makes you feel bad about yourself.

A to-do list is a powerful motivational tool if used properly. To find balance in your daily activities and to escape the enormous psychological weight and pressure that a to-do list can generate, it will serve you best to cut down your to-do list. A long list of things-to-do can be very overwhelming and cause you to worry unnecessarily.

Take a good look at your to-do list. How many items do you have written down to accomplish today: 20, 40, or more? A long list of things that needs to be done in one day usually points to a mind full of uncontrollable and discordant thoughts. I am not suggesting that it is wrong to want to accomplish many things in a day, but your ability to recognize important and urgent tasks will help you be more organized and prune down your list. So, go ahead and write down all the tasks that are popping up in your head. Now go through your list and pick out only the top five most important tasks that, if completed today, will give you the greatest sense of accomplishment. Those are the tasks that you should give your undivided attention. The rest are merely worrisome thoughts appearing as important things to get in your way of accomplishing what will give you joy and fulfillment.

Create Three Lists

Do not discard the rest of the items you took off your daily to-do list. Put them on a separate list. Ideally, you should have three lists. The first list for high-impact tasks that need to be done today, a second list for tasks that need to be accomplished within the current week, and the third list for relatively long-term goals – things that you need to get done within a month or more. When you split up your tasks into different lists, you save yourself the headache of worrying over things that can wait and use that energy and time on something more important and urgent.

Group Your Daily Tasks into Batches of Similar Tasks

Imagine that you have to jump from writing a 2,000-word article to doing the laundry. Then you have to have to edit your article, prepare lunch, and then respond to your emails. If you reorganize the tasks so that similar activities are performed following each other, it helps you flow easily from one task to the other without having to spend too much time and effort trying to mentally refocus on a new task. So, you could write your article, edit it, and respond to your emails, before doing the laundry and preparing lunch, for example.

Recognize the Difference between Important and Urgent Tasks

When you live your life thinking you don't have enough time, you are prone to develop anxiety. In other words, your life is filled with a sense of urgency – everything must be done right this red-hot minute or else your world will come crashing! That is living as if you are under a life-and-death threat, essentially stimulating the SNS.

If you take some time to ask how important a task is, you can then realistically determine whether it deserves to be handled urgently. Rather than trying to respond to urgent tasks, become deliberate about your responses by attending to important tasks instead. For example, when you get to work, instead of diving headlong into urgent tasks, go first for the important things. Plan what do you want to accomplish for the day and get to work on them before responding to other seemingly urgent matters. By working this way, you are deliberately removing yourself from the urge to respond to "urgent" stimuli, thereby increasing your chances of feeling fulfilled and satisfied with your accomplishments for that day.

Focus on Your Plans, Not Other's

What are the things you do in the first few minutes after you wake up in the morning or when you get to work? For many people, their activities when they wake up or get to work include:

- Check their inbox for emails.
- Check their phone for text messages or missed calls.
- Look up the social media for responses and reactions to their posts.
- Turn on the TV or read the newspaper for the current news (which is usually bad news).

These activities are likely to put you in a reactionary place – following other people's schedules and plans and ignoring yours (if at all you have a plan). In other words, you prime your mind to prioritize other people's agenda. You also set yourself up to start your day or working hours with negative news and unnecessary pressure. This is a sure path to unnecessary worry and anxiety.

Consciously resist the urge to grab your phone when you wake up in the morning. Refuse to dive into your inbox as soon as you get to work. Set aside at least 20 minutes of your day to plan what you want to accomplish for that day. This will give you a sense of direction and save you from deviating from your plan to do what others have set out for you.

Create Time for Focused Work

Whether you are working from home or not, or whether your work is taking care of the home, saving lives, or preparing your company's budget, you need to create time for focused work when you shut off all forms of distraction and pay undivided attention to what you do.

We live in a world that is increasingly filled with stimuli requiring your attention. Phones, TVs, tablets, and so on are not just mere distractions but also sources of stress and anxiety. When you allow yourself to be distracted by the plethora of stimuli in your environment, you get less done and end up pressuring yourself to be more productive in the remaining time you have left.

So, set aside around 40 to 50 minutes where you concentrate solely on just one task until you complete it. Cut off every distraction – shut the door, switch off your phone or put it on silent, turn off notifications on your browser, and put on your headphones (if you work better with music). When you are done with a task, take a 10-minute break to refocus your mind before taking on another task. Periods of intense mental and physical engagement (focused work) can make you get into the flow of things and increase your productivity. Getting things done properly also increases your satisfaction and happiness levels – a natural deterrent for anxiety.

Learn to Keep a Schedule

Creating a list of things to be done is one thing; doing them is another thing entirely. It is a lot easier to put things off to a later time than doing them when they are supposed to be done. But all that does is to put you under pressure to complete those tasks when time is running out. It is ill-advised to overwork yourself, but it is equally not healthy to put off until another time what you should do now.

Having a to-do list does not automatically translate into a productive use of your time, nor does it mean you are free from stressful thoughts. There are people with watertight schedules who still think and feel, "I am just not a productive person!"

Ask yourself the following questions when making a schedule or to-do list:

1. Have I included extra time for this activity just in case other activities spillover?
2. Am I allotting shorter periods for big tasks?

3. Have I factored in my playtime or am I just focused on work time alone?
4. Do I consider deadlines while creating slots for my tasks?
5. Am I conscious of things that still need to be done or just following a list regardless of deadlines?

When you make a schedule, stick with it unless it is unavoidably necessary to deviate from it. Remember that you are essentially trading your life for whatever you choose to do with your time. If you allow any and everything to steal your time, you are giving away an invaluable resource (time) that can never be regained, and you may as well not bother having a schedule.

Stay Calm If Things Pop Up

Regardless of how well you plan your day, sometimes things don't go as planned. Uncertainty cannot be ruled out. Fixating on everything going as planned is trying to fight uncertainty – a fight you will never win. Accept uncertainty; make up your mind that you'll do your very best to fulfill your promises, keep your appointments, accomplish your tasks, and do what is expected of you. But if some things happen that are out of your control, remain calm. Don't stress yourself over what you cannot control. Worrying over what "should have been" is self-defeating and counterproductive. Realize that, in real life, things pop up that you didn't plan for, and a lot of the time, these things that "pop up" disrupt even the best of our plans. The healthier option for you to take is to simply accept the situation and find a way around, under, or through it. Other times, you may have to completely shelve your initial plans and come up with something entirely different in the light of the new development. This is effective time and energy management instead of wasting time and energy worrying and increasing your chances of becoming stressed.

Find Out Where You Are Spending Your Time

What you spend most of your time doing can impact your stress level. Whether it is online or offline, what you spend your time doing will determine if you are using your most precious resource to be more productive or to hurt yourself.

A simple way to know if your time was well spent or not is to ask yourself how you felt while you were in a place you've been.

- Did you enjoy your time?
- Who did you interact with?
- Were they pushing your buttons or was it mostly an enjoyable interaction?
- Did you have to go out of your way to please them?

- Did you feel pressured into conforming or were you encouraged to be yourself?
- Did you feel a sense of accomplishment after the interaction or did you feel drained?
- Would you like to go back there or do you dread going back there?
- Do you spend time there out of habit or because you feel truly great being there?

When you are honest about where you enjoy spending your time, you will dissociate yourself from places that are likely to trigger anxious thoughts in you.

Make Time for Yourself

There's one constant factor in all of your activities, and that is you. You can't keep the appointment, pay the bills, stay physically and mentally fit, and be productive at work if you are taken out of the equation. So, while you are busy running around trying to accomplish everything on your to-do list, remember to include some quality time to take care of yourself.

This could mean spending quality time with loved ones daily, taking time off from work for some vacation with your family, or pampering yourself with a massage. For some people, letting go and simply swinging from a hammock doing nothing but relaxing for 10 minutes is a scary idea! They have convinced themselves that their world could go up in smoke if they are not on top of the situation 100% of the time. But that type of thinking will only make you stressed up. Stop thinking that your kids, spouse, job, or whatever is important to you will come to a grinding halt if you take a few moments off to care for yourself. You are as equally important as these things you give your time to; in fact, you are top priority! If you don't take care of yourself, who will?

Here are some quick tips to help you make time for yourself.

1. Try to define why you need more time for yourself. You are more likely to make time for yourself if you attach a specific goal to it.
2. Delegate some tasks whether at home or work.
3. Think of tasks that you can outsource without compromising quality.
4. Figure out things you can do less of.
5. Don't compromise rest. Leave your work at work.

Chapter 5: Therapeutic and Clinical Treatment

Implementing the steps outlined in the previous chapters can effectively handle anxiety. However, some anxiety cases will require that you see a doctor for clinical treatment, visit a therapist for psychotherapy, or a combination of both. Also, if the idea of practicing some of the steps in the previous chapters sounds too spooky for you, you could opt for therapy or clinical treatment. In this final chapter, I shall outline a few tips on treating anxiety with therapy and medications.

Therapy

If you have any anxiety disorder or any mental health disorder, I highly recommend that you see a therapist. A therapist is qualified to guide you through a recovery process and can be the shoulder you need when your resolve is not as strong as it needs to be. Your therapist can determine the best treatment and course of action for you. A therapist will also introduce you to tools that you can use even after your treatment to improve the quality of your life. These tools include:

- Progressive Muscle Relaxation
- Relaxation Breathing
- Pleasant Activity Scheduling
- Cognitive Restructuring
- Successive Approximation
- Journaling
- Reframing Negative Thoughts
- Cognitive Behavioral Therapy (CBT) Worksheets to help you in the recovery process

However, if you are sure that what you have is everyday anxiety (mild anxiety) or the "almost anxious" level of worry (moderate anxiety), then you can administer therapy on your own. Also, it is possible that you are not able to afford a therapist or a therapist is not accessible in your location. I'll recommend that you use CBT techniques to help you in your recovery process. Keep in mind that you will need extra commitment to motivate and advise yourself if you are using CBT on your own. Also, note that this may not be a suitable choice for you if you have a chronic case of anxiety disorder.

The Self-Option CBT Guidelines

Here are a few guidelines to help you administer CBT by yourself.

1. Keep your motivation up by reading self-help books that align with your goals. Don't just buy books because they have nice-sounding titles. Be sure that you buy and read books that have the right tone for you.
2. Give enough consideration to sound research. Make sure that the books and materials you consult for CBT are based on proven scientific research.
3. Commit to the process. The fact that you are doing this by yourself doesn't mean you should go through your therapy sessions halfheartedly or that you should rush the process. Avoid squeezing your therapy session in between tight schedules.
4. Resist the temptation to skip parts of your therapy program because you feel you already know them. Go through with your program religiously as if you are attending a session with a therapist. Full commitment is what will bring about the results you desire.

Changing Your Lifestyle to Regain Control of Your Life

Taking back control of your life from anxiety and panic attacks will require you to make the following cognitive and behavioral changes.

Cognitive Techniques

- Observe your thoughts without judgment and then try to determine whether they are logical. This will mean that you assume the position of an impartial umpire as you assess your thoughts on each subject that easily drag you down the path of worry.
- Observe the connection between your thoughts and feelings because your behavior is largely dependent on how you feel.
- Determine if your thoughts and feelings are correct, rational, and based in reality. Do you have any concrete evidence to prove their correctness? Subjecting your thoughts and feelings about situations to critical questioning will bring to light their rationality or otherwise.

- Finally, replace irrational and baseless thoughts with more realistic ones. The more unhelpful thoughts you can challenge and replace, the better you'll feel, and ultimately, the better you'll behave.

Behavioral Techniques

- Get in the habit of doing the things you love doing. When you do, you boost your sense of accomplishment and feel better about yourself. Go to places where you enjoy going and engage in fun activities to improve your overall emotional state of being.

- When you do something that makes you feel good, acknowledge it. Doing so can strengthen neural connections between your emotions, thoughts, and actions.

- Become deliberate about your daily activities. The more aware you become of your activities, the more you increase your chances of responding consciously.

- Break down your goals and daily activities into smaller bits. This will remove unnecessary stress that can arise from feeling overwhelmed by the size of your tasks and goals.

Quality Sleep Decreases Worry and Anxiety

Perhaps one of the simplest forms of therapy for anxiety is quality sleep. Maintaining a good sleeping habit can decrease your chances of falling prey to anxiety disorders.

One train of thought can deprive you of quality sleep. Your sleeping environment and bedtime behavior can have the same effect. Nighttime usually has fewer activities to keep your attention distracted from worries, which means your chances of ruminating over situations and issues are greater at night. But you can tip the scale in your favor if you create a conducive sleeping environment. Here are a few tips for developing good bedtime rituals and how to make your sleeping space conducive for sleep.

1. Create a bedtime routine that can put you in a relaxed state before you fall asleep. You can begin your bedtime ritual an hour before you sleep. Be consistent about the routine so that each time you start it, your body is queued up for sleep. The ritual or routine can include taking warm baths, reading a page or two from a book that does not stimulate conflict in your thoughts, practice yoga, or meditation. Make sure that your bedtime activity is low-

key and stress-free.

2. Troubling discussions and arguments before bedtime can hinder quality sleep. Avoid them as much as possible especially before you go to sleep.

3. Endeavor to make your sleeping space or bedroom as conducive as possible and optimized for a good night's sleep. If you have a television in your bedroom or sleeping space, switch it off long before your bedtime. Make sure the noise level in your bedroom is low, the lights are turned off or dimmed, and the temperature is perfect. Make your bed as comfortable as possible.

4. Your body should be getting ready to sleep at night and not getting ready to begin fresh work. Keep away from eating or taking caffeine right before bedtime.

5. Make sure that you sleep for at least 7 hours per night which is the recommended sleep time for adults (National Sleep Foundation, 2015). Getting enough night sleep allows your body to rejuvenate.

6. No matter what, do not snooze your alarm because the usual snooze time is not enough to give you time for quality sleep. It will only annoy you again when you are starting to enjoy your second round of sleep. When your alarm goes off, get up and begin your day – that's the

reason you set an alarm in the first place. Besides, sleeping for the recommended sleep time would give you enough sleep such that you don't need to snooze your alarm. Always make sure that your alarm clock is kept far away from your bed so that you have to get up from bed to stop it from ringing.

7. Create time for having short naps during the day for about 20 minutes. Sleeping in the day time for short periods can energize your brain and help you wake up refreshed.

8. Blue light such as the ones given off by smartphones and computer screens can reduce the stimulation of hormones responsible for making you fall asleep. Exposing yourself to blue light tricks your brain into assuming it's still day time. So, keep your smartphones and laptops away from your bed. Your bed should be meant for rest, relaxation, and sleep, and not for chatting into the night or getting a head start on the next day's work.

9. The circadian rhythm is your body's internal clock that aligns itself with sunrise and sunset. Following a regular sleep schedule ensures that your circadian rhythm remains intact. On the other hand, if you keep shifting your bedtime, you interrupt the circadian rhythm and

your internal clock. This is why you should form the habit of going to bed almost at the same time every night. This is also the reason you should keep your afternoon nap short so that it doesn't mess up your internal clock and keep you up late into the night.

10. Empty your bladder and bowels before going to bed to avoid waking up several times during the night. Bathroom visits can disrupt your sleep and leave you grumpy in the morning.

Medication for Anxiety and Panic Attacks

You may opt to see a doctor instead of a therapist for whatever reason. Mostly, people anxiety disorders may not have the patience to go through therapy; they want results and they want them now! As good as anxiety medications are, they may have some unpleasant side effects. Equally, taking the time to go through CBT can help you make a lifestyle change once and for all. That is to say, you will be able to handle subsequent cases of anxiety issues should you experience a relapse. But with medication, if you experience a relapse, you will have to use the medications again. This can lead to overdependence on drugs.

Nevertheless, here are some common medications that can be

used in treating anxiety disorders. I have also outlined their possible side effects. If for whatever reason you choose to stop using any medication for anxiety, I strongly suggest that you see a qualified doctor before doing so. Abruptly stopping medications for anxiety can result in very unpleasant side effects.

1. **Benzodiazepines for Anxiety**

    These are the commonest types of medication prescribed for anxiety. They are also known as tranquilizers. Benzodiazepines have a way of slowing your nervous system so that you can relax both mentally and physically. Typically, they work very quickly to bring about relief. But they are easily addictive and therefore not recommended for long-term use.

    The following are the different types of benzodiazepines:

    - Ativan (lorazepam)
    - Klonopin (clonazepam)
    - Valium (diazepam)
    - Xanax (alprazolam)

    Common side effects include:

    - Drowsiness
    - Dizziness

- Poor balance or coordination
- Slurred speech
- Trouble concentrating
- Memory problems
- Confusion
- Upset stomach
- Headache
- Blurred vision

2. **Beta-Blockers**

Beta-blockers are typically used for treating heart problems and high blood pressure, but they can also be prescribed for anxiety. Beta-blockers prevent the effect of the stress hormone responsible for the fight-or-flight response, essentially controlling rapid heart rate, sweating, shaking, and so on. However, emotional symptoms, such as worry, are not controlled. This makes beta-blockers most suitable for social phobias.

Beta blockers include the following drugs:

- Propranolol (Inderal)
- Atenolol (Tenormin)

Common side effects include:

- Dizziness

- Sleepiness
- Weakness
- Fatigue
- Nausea
- Headaches
- Constipation
- Diarrhea

3. **Buspirone (BuSpar)**

This is a milder tranquilizer and takes about 2 weeks for its effects to be felt. Buspirone works by decreasing dopamine and increasing serotonin in the brain. Generally, its effects are minimal compared to benzodiazepines. However, it seems to be more suitable for generalized anxiety disorder (GAD) than other types of anxiety disorders.

Common side effects include:

- Nausea
- Headaches
- Dizziness
- Drowsiness
- Weight gain
- Upset stomach

- Constipation
- Nervousness
- Diarrhea
- Dry mouth

4. **SSRI Antidepressants for Anxiety**

Antidepressants are originally prescribed for depression but can also be used for treating anxiety. SSRIs (Selective Serotonin Reuptake Inhibitors) are more suitable for ongoing treatment of chronic anxiety problems. They can be used in the treatment of panic disorders, post-traumatic stress disorder (PTSD), generalized anxiety disorder (GAD), social anxiety disorder, and obsessive-compulsive disorder (OCD).

SSRIs commonly used for anxiety include:

- Celexa
- Lexapro
- Paxil
- Prozac
- Zoloft

Common side effects include:

- Fatigue
- Nausea

- Agitation
- Drowsiness
- Weight gain
- Diarrhea
- Insomnia
- Sexual dysfunction
- Nervousness
- Headaches
- Dry mouth
- Increased sweating

Questions to Ask Yourself

Before you opt for medications, consider the following questions:

1. Is medication the best option for your worries and anxiety problems?
2. Can you endure the unpleasant side effects of the medications in return for instant relief?
3. Are there other treatments available for anxiety that don't involve medications?
4. Would I be able to be patient to follow through with CBT?
5. Would I be willing to combine medication and CBT?
6. What other self-help techniques can I use to reduce my anxiety?

7. Do I really have an anxiety problem or do I have an underlying health condition?

Questions to Ask Your Doctor

Consider asking your doctor the following questions before settling for medications:

1. In what way will medication improve my anxiety problem?
2. What are the common side effects of the prescribed drugs?
3. What drinks and foods do I need to avoid during treatment?
4. Will this drug have any negative impact on my health if I am currently taking other prescription medications?
5. How long will I have to be under treatment?
6. Would I have a difficult time withdrawing from this medication?
7. If I stop taking the drug, would my anxiety problems return?

Herbal Supplements for Treating Anxiety

Supplements may help to ease some symptoms of anxiety, but

they certainly are not meant to replace prescribed medication and therapies. Make sure to speak with your doctor before using any herbal supplements for anxiety. Generally, supplements for anxiety are not recommended for pregnant women, young children, and adults who are over 65 years.

Herbal supplements are usually in the form of tea, extracts, tinctures, or capsules. Here are a few of the most common ones used in the treatment of anxiety.

1. **Kava Kava**

   This is a plant found in the Pacific Islands. It is traditionally used as a calming tonic. It may help in boosting your body's natural ability to manage anxiety.

2. **Valerian**

   This is typically a sleep remedy but may also help with easing symptoms associated with anxiety.

3. **St. John's Wort**

   Typically, this is used as an herb for the treatment of depression. But it can also be used for reducing anxiety, especially depression-related anxiety.

4. **Passionflower**

   The use of St. John's Wort for anxiety seems to be riddled

with controversy. But when combined with other herbs, it may be more effective. Passionflower is one such herb that, when combined with St. John's Wort, may produce a better result.

Two other methods that can be used for treating anxiety include:

1. Aromatherapy – the use of aromatic plant extracts and essential oils for treatment.
2. Acupuncture – the use of special needles on the specific parts of the body for the treatment of mental and physical conditions.

However, it is important to speak with your doctor first if you are interested in using these methods. For acupuncture, make sure that you consult a licensed acupuncturist.

Conclusion

Worrying about anxiety doesn't make it go away any faster! So, your first step in recovery is to let go of the need to make your anxiety go away immediately. On some deep level, people who resort to illicit drugs and substances to make them forget their worries are seeking quick fixes. But soon enough, the effect of these substances (whether legal or not) wear off and they come out of their altered states of consciousness where they have enjoyed temporal pleasure and freedom from bothersome thoughts. For some, the pain of facing reality is unimaginable, so they return to these substances again and again until it becomes an addiction. Instead of dealing with one problem – worry – they now have two major problems: anxiety and addiction.

Remember that it took a lot of time for your worrisome thoughts and feelings of anxiety to reach the level of a bad habit and a health challenge. It will also take some time for you to get rid of the habit and recover from the health challenges, so be patient. Even if you use CBT, prescription medication, or both to treat anxiety, you still have to be patient so that you don't become over-dependent on prescription medication.

There is always a time lag between being "almost anxious" and an anxiety disorder, as we have seen in Chapter 1. That would be the ideal time to deal with your anxiety issues by applying the practical steps described in this book. However, even if you are experiencing the normal, everyday worry or you have slipped into the clinical anxiety level, it is still helpful to follow these practical techniques until they become your new mental habit. Remember that, just as it takes constant negative self-talk to get you into a predominantly worried state, it also takes constant positive self-talk to put you in a good frame of mind. This may not change your circumstances or make your problems go away instantly, but it can make you begin to look at your situation from a different and more productive perspective. So, instead of shooting yourself in the foot in the process of worrying, positive self-talk can open you up to ideas that would have been otherwise closed-off from your worried and negative mindset.

Some of the techniques described in this book may be foreign to you, sound too religious, or somewhat esoteric. For someone entirely new to these ideas, practicing them can also be tiring, especially the breathing, meditation, and mindfulness techniques. It is normal to feel weird (and even frustrated) about these techniques at first, but I encourage you to stick with them. The benefits outweigh any temporal perceptual and physical discomfort you may experience at first. Do not be afraid that the practices will turn you into some social misfit – you don't have to practice them in the presence of anyone, nor are they meant to influence your religious inclinations in any way. Your personal beliefs are entirely your business; the techniques in this book only seek to help you get rid of limiting beliefs that can inhibit your daily mental and physical performances.

Finally, practice, practice, practice – that is the surest way to gain mastery over worry and anxiety.

References

American Psychological Association. (2019). Anxiety. Retrieved from https://www.apa.org/topics/anxiety/

Ami, T. (2019). 6 Yoga poses that help alleviate anxiety. Retrieved from https://www.doyouyoga.com/6-yoga-poses-that-help-alleviate-anxiety-38992/

Andre, C. (2019). Proper breathing brings better health. Retrieved from https://www.scientificamerican.com/article/proper-breathing-brings-better-health/

Aylett, E. Small, N. and Bower, P. (2018). Exercise in the treatment of clinical anxiety in general practice – a systematic review and meta-analysis. Retrieved from https://bmchealthservres.biomedcentral.com/articles/10.1186/s12913-018-3313-5

Biostrap Team. (2017). Hacking your parasympathetic nervous system. Retrieved from https://biostrap.com/blog/hacking-your-parasympathetic-nervous-system/

Black, D. S., PhD, MPH, et al. (2015). Mindfulness meditation and improvement in sleep quality and daytime impairment among older adults with sleep disturbances: A randomized clinical trial. Retrieved from https://jamanetwork.com/journals/jamainternalmedicine/fullarticle/2110998

Carlson, L. E. PhD, et al. (2014). Mindfulness-based cancer recovery and supportive-expressive therapy maintain telomere length relative to controls in distressed breast cancer survivors. Retrieved from https://onlinelibrary.wiley.com/doi/full/10.1002/cncr.29063

Dunn, J. (2017). Negative self-talk: 9 ways to silence your inner critic. Retrieved from https://www.huffpost.com/entry/negative-self-talk-think-positive_n_3009832

Diffen. (2014). Parasympathetic vs. sympathetic nervous system. Retrieved from https://www.diffen.com/difference/Parasympathetic_nervous_system_vs_Sympathetic_nervous_system

Elmer, J. (2018). 5 Ways to stop spiraling negative thoughts from taking control. Retrieved from https://www.healthline.com/health/mental-health/stop-automatic-negative-thoughts#7

Gotter, A. (2019). 8 Breathing exercises to try when you feel anxious. Retrieved from https://www.healthline.com/health/breathing-exercises-for-anxiety#yoga-breaths

Hanson, R. Ph.D. (2007). Relaxed and content (part two): Activating the parasympathetic wing of your nervous system. Retrieved from https://www.rickhanson.net/relaxed-content-part-two-activating-parasympathetic-wing-nervous-system/

Harvard Health Publishing. (2011). Understanding the stress response. Chronic activation of this survival mechanism impairs health. Retrieved from https://www.health.harvard.edu/staying-healthy/understanding-the-stress-response

Healthlink BC. (2017). Anxiety: Stop negative thoughts. Retrieved from https://www.healthlinkbc.ca/health-topics/uf9897

Hoehn-Saric R. and McLeod DR. (2000). Anxiety and arousal: Physiological changes and their perception. Retrieved from https://www.ncbi.nlm.nih.gov/pubmed/11163423

Hurley, T. (2018). Activating the parasympathetic nervous system to decrease stress and anxiety. Retrieved from https://canyonvista.com/activating-parasympathetic-nervous-system/

International Journal of Behavioral Medicine. (2015). Positive associations of dispositional mindfulness with cardiovascular health: The new England family study. Retrieved from https://link.springer.com/article/10.1007/s12529-014-9448-9

King, Anna Lucia S., et al. (2010). Nomophobia: The mobile phone in panic disorder with agoraphobia: Reducing phobias or worsening of dependence? Retrieved from https://journals.lww.com/cogbehavneurol/Abstract/2010/03000/Nomophobia__The_Mobile_Phone_in_Panic_Disorder.10.aspx

Marques, L. Ph.D. (2018). Do I have anxiety or worry: What's the difference? Retrieved from https://www.health.harvard.edu/blog/do-i-have-anxiety-or-worry-whats-the-difference-2018072314303

Mawer, R. (2018). 17 Proven tips to sleep better at night. Retrieved from https://www.healthline.com/nutrition/17-tips-to-sleep-better

Medical Daily. (2013). Mindfulness meditation reduces pain associated with arthritis, asthma. Retrieved from https://www.medicaldaily.com/mindfulness-meditation-reduces-pain-associated-arthritis-asthma-244309

Medical Daily. (2016). Mindfulness vs meditation: The difference between these two pathways to well-being and peace of mind. Retrieved from https://www.medicaldaily.com/mindfulness-meditation-differences-377346

Mental Help. (2019). Visualization and Guided Imagery Techniques for Stress Reduction. Retrieved from https://www.mentalhelp.net/stress/visualization-and-guided-imagery-techniques-for-stress-reduction/

National Sleep Foundation. (2015). National sleep foundation recommends new sleep times. Retrieved from https://www.sleepfoundation.org/press-release/national-sleep-foundation-recommends-new-sleep-times

National Institute of Health. (2008). A bidirectional relationship between anxiety and depression, and insomnia? A prospective study in the general population. Retrieved from https://www.ncbi.nlm.nih.gov/pubmed/18374745

National Institute of Health. (2017). Validity of the associated symptom criteria for generalized anxiety disorder: Observations from the Singapore mental health study. Retrieved from https://www.ncbi.nlm.nih.gov/pubmed/27805985

National Institute of Health. (2017). Effects of gratitude meditation on neural network functional connectivity and brain-heart coupling. Retrieved from https://www.ncbi.nlm.nih.gov/pmc/articles/PMC5506019/

NHS. (2019). Selective mutism. Retrieved from https://www.nhs.uk/conditions/selective-mutism/

Psychology Today. (2015). 7 Scientifically proven benefits of gratitude. Retrieved from https://www.psychologytoday.com/intl/blog/what-mentally-strong-people-dont-do/201504/7-scientifically-proven-benefits-gratitude

Robinson, L. et al (2019). How to stop worrying. Retrieved from https://www.helpguide.org/articles/anxiety/how-to-stop-worrying.htm

Science Daily. (2014). Mindfulness intervention boosts brain activation for healthy pleasures. Retrieved from https://www.sciencedaily.com/releases/2014/12/141205142434.htm

Scott, E. (2019). Top 10 stress-relieving hobbies. Retrieved from https://www.verywellmind.com/top-stress-reliever-hobbies-3144592

Sharma, A. et al. (2006). Exercise for mental health. Retrieved from https://www.ncbi.nlm.nih.gov/pmc/articles/PMC1470658/

Smith, M., Robinson, L. and Segal, J. (2019). Anxiety medication. Retrieved from https://www.helpguide.org/articles/anxiety/anxiety-medication.htm

Star, K. Ph.D. (2019). How yoga can help ease anxiety and panic disorder symptoms. Retrieved from https://www.verywellmind.com/yoga-for-panic-disorder-2584114

White, A. (2018). Try this: 25 Supplements for anxiety. Retrieved from https://www.healthline.com/health/anxiety/supplements-for-anxiety#takeaway

Yoga Journal. (2019). Yoga for anxiety. Retrieved from https://www.yogajournal.com/poses/yoga-by-benefit/anxiety

Printed in Great Britain
by Amazon

35570660R00086